Thieme

Encyclopedia of Football Medicine

Volume 1: Trauma and Medical Emergencies

Jonny Gordon, MBChB, MSc, MFSEM FRCEM, FRCP
Consultant in Emergency Medicine
Queen Elizabeth University Hospital
Glasgow, UK
Team Doctor
Scottish National Football Team

Anna Nordström, MD, Phd
Specialist in Rehabilitation Medicine
Northern University Hospital
Associate Professor in Sports Medicine
Umeå University
Umeå, Sweden

66 illustrations

Thieme
Stuttgart • New York • Delhi • Rio de Janeiro

Library of Congress Cataloging-in-Publication Data is available from the publisher.

Thieme Publishers New York
333 Seventh Avenue, New York, NY 10001, USA
+1 800 782 3488, customerservice@thieme.com

Thieme Publishers Stuttgart
Rüdigerstrasse 14, 70469 Stuttgart, Germany
+1 800 782 3488, customerservice@thieme.com

Thieme Publishers Delhi
A-12, Second Floor, Sector-2, Noida-201301
Uttar Pradesh, India
+91 120 45 566 00, customerservice@thieme.in

Thieme Publishers Rio, Thieme Publicações Ltda.
Edifício Rodolpho de Paoli, 25º andar
Av. Nilo Peçanha, 50 – Sala 2508
Rio de Janeiro 20020-906 Brasil
+55 21 3172 2297 / +55 21 3172 1896

Cover design: Thieme Publishing Group
Photographs – Getty Images, UEFA
(All football images including the cover.)
Typesetting by Ditech Process Solutions, India

Printed in Germany, CPI Books in Leck

ISBN 978-3-13-220321-1 23456

Also available as an e-book:
eISBN 978-3-13-220331-0

Important note: Medicine is an ever-changing science undergoing continual development. Research and clinical experience are continually expanding our knowledge, in particular our knowledge of proper treatment and drug therapy. Insofar as this book mentions any dosage or application, readers may rest assured that the authors, editors, and publishers have made every effort to ensure that such references are in accordance with **the state of knowledge at the time of production of the book.**

Nevertheless, this does not involve, imply, or express any guarantee or responsibility on the part of the publishers with respect to any dosage instructions and forms of applications stated in the book. **Every user is requested to examine carefully** the manufacturers' leaflets accompanying each drug and to check, if necessary in consultation with a physician or specialist, whether the dosage schedules mentioned therein or the contraindications stated by the manufacturers differ from the statements made in the present book. Such examination is particularly important with drugs that either are rarely used or have been newly released on the market. Every dosage schedule or every form of application used is entirely at the user's own risk and responsibility. The authors and publishers request every user to report to the publishers any discrepancies or inaccuracies noticed. If errors in this work are found after publication, errata will be posted at www.thieme.com on the product description page.

Some of the product names, patents, and registered designs referred to in this book are in fact registered trademarks or proprietary names even though specific reference to this fact is not always made in the text. Therefore, the appearance of a name without designation as proprietary is not to be construed as a representation by the publisher that it is in the public domain.

FSC www.fsc.org
MIX
Papier aus verantwortungsvollen Quellen
FSC® C083411

Contents

Foreword

As modern football has progressed in recent years, the role of the team doctor has become ever more important to the success of its teams, not only in protecting the health and fitness of players, but also in providing a comprehensive and scientifically advanced medical support service. The role of the doctor now encompasses medical team planning and management, first aid techniques, injury prevention, health promotion, rehabilitation, and many more areas, meaning that the doctor is now one of the key positions in any successful football team.

As an organization, UEFA always seeks to further scientific research and to provide the best standards of medical care for players, and these books bring together some of the most eminent practitioners in all aspects of the now very specific domain of football medicine. All areas of the modern football doctor's toolkit are covered with advice on advanced treatment techniques, management of the medical team, and best practice in all areas of the doctor's role. UEFA's many years of work in football medicine and the extensive experience of the chapter authors make this an indispensable text for any doctor wishing to work in the field.

As we look toward the future and the further development and dissemination of football-specific medical expertise, I hope that this book will serve you well as a reference guide in a sport that is now so technically and scientifically advanced to be almost unrecognizable from the one within which I started my career.

I hope that you will enjoy this book and the book series.

Michel D'Hooghe, MD
Bruges, Belgium

Preface

The first volume of the *Encyclopedia of Football Medicine*, entitled *Trauma and Medical Emergencies*, instructs on advanced techniques for managing the treatment of serious and life-threatening on-field injury. The content of this first volume was initially developed as the course manual of the first workshop of the UEFA Football Doctor Education Programme in Vienna in 2012. The workshop and course manual were highly appreciated by the national team doctors who attended the course, as emergency medicine is an area they are not regularly confronted with.

Dr. Jonny Gordon was contracted to run and develop this workshop for UEFA as the Trauma and Medical Emergencies expert. He developed Chapters 1 to 5 of this book, covering the different steps and scenarios of emergencies that can be expected on the pitch. Prof. Anna Nordström focuses in Chapter 6 on the specificity of head injuries in football. This chapter was added on in a later stage, following the concussion incidences at the 2014 World Cup in Brazil. It was initially presented and included in the manual of the third workshop of the Football Doctor Education Programme in 2015; however, due to its similar content to Volume 1, we decided to include it here.

The aim of this manual and the UEFA medical course is to familiarize clinicians with a structured system of assessment that can be applied to any footballer regardless of the presenting condition, and to give clinicians the confidence to put this system into practice. The goal is to attain a generic standard to allow the best possible care to be provided to our players.

This book starts by introducing the first crucial steps to know in a medical emergency on the pitch, going over the initial assessments such as the airway, the cervical spine, breathing, circulation, and disability. It then moves on to the specific cardiac arrest and chocking situation, taking the doctors step by step through the European Resuscitation Council (ERC) Guidelines 2015. In the first chapter, a variety of medical emergencies are presented which football doctors might face during their career while explaining the diagnoses and treatments of these medical emergencies. These medical emergencies include anaphylaxis, asthma, seizures, and diabetic emergencies. In the following chapter, trauma emergencies are covered, such as spinal injuries, head and facial traumas, chest traumas, abdominal traumas, pelvic traumas, and limb and lower limb traumas. It concludes with more general medical managements of possible emergencies on the pitch, such as analgesia and anesthesia, wound management, and the medical kit to carry. The last chapter of this book explains the risk of head injuries and especially concussions in football by going over the definitions, causes and mechanisms, evaluation and management via different baseline tests, follow-up evaluation and management, the risks in recovery, and the issue of repetitive concussions.

Chapter 1

First Steps

Jonny Gordon

Having a sound framework and system of assessment is the cornerstone to ensuring a complete and thorough assessment of the seriously injured or unwell player.

It is unlikely that you will be faced with a sudden death during your time looking after a football team. It is, however, likely that you will be involved in treating players who have sustained life-threatening medical or trauma emergencies. Having a structured process to fall back on when under pressure is a vital aspect of providing sound clinical care.

Irrespective of cause, the initial assessment of any "critical" patient utilizes the same ABC system. The assessment, recognition, and treatment of life-threatening conditions must take place in a structured manner. The only variance between medical and trauma emergencies is the need in trauma to control the cervical spine while dealing with the airway.

Unless specifically ruled out, such as in an observed, witnessed collapse without trauma, the cervical spine should always be assumed to be injured.

The mechanism of injury provides us with vital information as to the likely extent of injury to the player:

- Two footballers clashing heads and then falling to the ground clearly raises the possibility of a cervical spine injury as well as a head injury.
- A player who rises to make a header, clashes with the goalkeeper, and flips over, landing on their back or side, may sustain life-threatening chest, abdominal, or pelvic injuries as well as potential spine and head injuries.
- Two players who collide while sliding in for a 50:50 tackle may sustain multiple and differing traumatic forces, such as direct impact in addition to rotational twisting forces to the limbs. Injury may occur anywhere from the foot to the head.

In these quickly occurring clashes, the actual mechanism may be unclear to the medic watching at pitchside, so a cervical spine injury should again be assumed until a structured assessment has been completed. In many cases, this may be achieved by simply questioning the player, followed by palpation and then gentle movement of the cervical spine. In others (especially where there is a "distracting injury"), full immobilization may be necessary and assessment deferred until the player has been completely removed from the field.

1.1 Framework for Initial Assessment

Regardless of the injury, each aspect of the framework (**Fig. 1.1**) must be considered, assessed, and, if necessary, treated before moving on to the next.

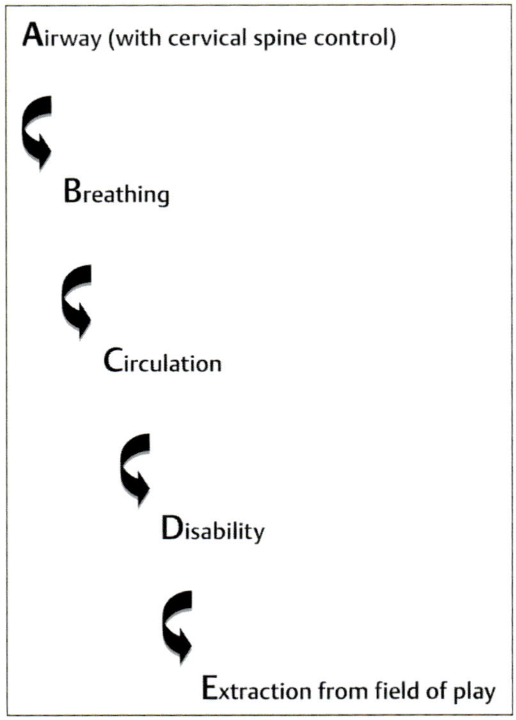

Fig. 1.1 Aspects of the framework for initial assessment, in the order they should be performed.

It may seem unnecessary to consider assessing the airway in a player who has twisted his ankle, but it should be an automatic response and the first question asked when dealing with any player on the pitch should be: "Were you hurt in any other way when you fell?"

Similarly, it is highly dangerous to focus on the nuances of the neurophysiological assessment of a footballer who has sustained a head injury if you do not give due consideration to the assessment of his potential cervical spine injury.

Put simply, as long as you always consider the possibility of more significant problems and are not immediately distracted by the gaping head wound or the ankle pointing the wrong way, then you are unlikely to miss more significant pathology.

We shall take each step of the framework and break it down in terms of assessment, potential problems to be looked for, and management.

The entire focus of the initial assessment is to keep things simple, not complicated. It could be argued that the only two items of kit required by a team doctor running onto a football pitch are gauze swabs and gloves. Simple maneuvers will allow you to treat the airway, protect the cervical spine, and assess breathing, circulation, and disability. Direct pressure via swabs will stop the vast majority of bleeding.

Everything else can be addressed in the dressing room, or in an ambulance if necessary.

The player's well-being must be the number one priority, as difficult as it may be to convey this to the manager who needs to know whether to substitute the player or not.

1.2 Airway

The airway can become compromised due to either primary or secondary trauma.

Primary Trauma. Trauma to the face, head, or neck can result in bleeding, bruising, or swelling that can make it physically difficult to shift air through the nasopharynx or oropharynx, the laryngopharynx, and into the lungs.

Secondary Trauma. Injury resulting in a decreased conscious level (usually assessed by either the Alert, Verbal, Pain, Unresponsive [AVPU] or Glasgow Coma Scale [GCS] scoring systems described on page 11) can seriously compromise the airway via an obtundation of the airway reflexes. In this situation, the anatomical structures of the airway may not be directly affected. However, the combination of a direct or primary injury to the airway (e.g., broken teeth or mandible) in association with a decreased GCS score significantly increases the risks of airway compromise and requires immediate action.

1.2.1 Airway Assessment and Management

The airway is best assessed by asking the simple question: "Are you ok?" As basic as this may seem, the information conveyed lets you know immediately that the player has a patent airway with which to shift air in and out to answer you. The rate at which they speak may suggest whether their breathing is affected or not. It indicates that blood pressure (BP) is sufficient to perfuse their brain, and it may also give an indication of the verbal and motor components of their GCS.

If the player does not respond, or the answer is inappropriate, vague, or confused, it is essential that both the airway and the cervical spine are assessed and protected. The easiest way to do this is to kneel beside the player and gently support the head in a neutral position in relation to the neck. The head should be held so that it is neither flexed nor extended upon the cervical spine.

Assessment of the airway and breathing should be done almost as one. If the player does not respond to the initial "Are you ok?", an airway-opening maneuver should be used and airway adjuncts administered as necessary.

The look, listen, and feel approach is then applied as described in more detail under the Breathing section later in the chapter.

Management of the airway can be divided into four sections:

- Airway-opening maneuvers.
- Basic airway adjuncts.
- Advanced airway adjuncts.
- Surgical airways.

Airway-Opening Maneuvers

Jaw Thrust

The jaw thrust should be used in any patient who has an obstructed airway when an injury to the cervical spine cannot be excluded. In trauma, this is the best method to relieve an airway obstruction because it can be carried out while still maintaining control over the cervical spine. In an obtunded player, the tongue can fall backward causing a soft-tissue obstruction to the oropharynx.

Technique. By simply placing the index finger of each hand directly under the angle of the mandible and lifting directly upward, the tongue is moved anteriorly away from the posterior pharynx, allowing airflow to be restored (**Fig. 1.2**).

Head Tilt and Chin Lift

The head tilt and chin lift can only be used in a patient who has an obstructed airway once an injury to the cervical spine has definitely been excluded. This technique is **contraindicated in trauma** as it requires movement of the head from a neutral position with the possible result of overflexion or extension of the neck and worsening of any spinal injury.

Technique. One hand is placed on the player's forehead. The other hand is placed with the thumb resting just below the lower lip and the index and middle fingers underneath the chin in the midline. The head is gently extended (so that the player is looking upward) and the chin is gently pulled forward in an anterior direction. Again, the tongue is moved anteriorly away from the posterior pharynx to allow increased airflow (**Fig. 1.3**).

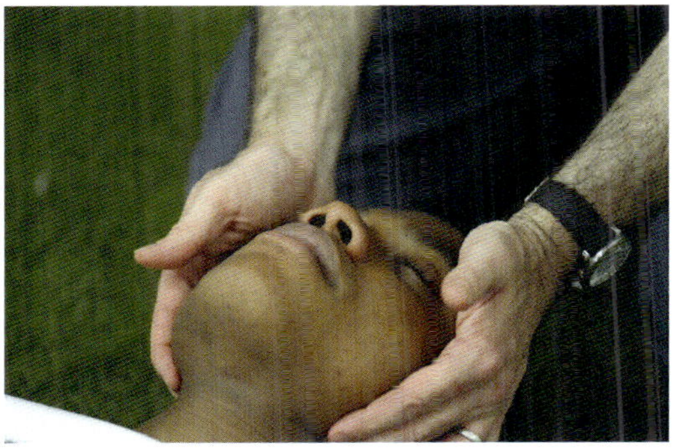

Fig. 1.2 Jaw thrust. Note that even with two people, the jaw thrust is the preferred technique to open the airway in a trauma situation.

These techniques should be sufficient in the majority of cases to open the airway and allow you to assess breathing.
If the airway cannot be controlled, i.e., it remains obstructed, airway adjuncts will be required.

Basic Airway Adjuncts

Oropharyngeal Airway (Guedel)

This firm plastic device is designed to fit into the airway and assist in helping to pull the tongue forward from the posterior pharyngeal wall.
The advantages of this kit are that it is cheap, readily available, portable, and can in most cases be used relatively easily. However, **if it is wrongly sized, or care is not taken when placing it, it may stimulate the gag reflex and cause the player to vomit.**
The Guedel comes in a range of sizes and is usually sized by measuring from the angle of the mandible to the front incisors (**Fig. 1.4a**).
It is placed upside down into the mouth and then rotated 180 degrees to lie with the plastic flange at the lips. If it keeps protruding from the lips after you have placed it, then consider resizing (**Fig. 1.4b**).

Nasopharyngeal Airway

The nasopharyngeal airway (NPA) is another adjunct commonly used to help airflow through the pharynx. It is made of soft plastic and can be used either in isolation or in conjunction with the Guedel airway. In principle, it should not be used when treating head injuries where there is a risk or signs suggestive of a base of skull fracture, as it may be incorrectly placed and find its way through the fracture and into the skull base. This is a recognized complication, though exceptionally rare. If it is the only airway adjunct available to you and you require one to support the airway as all other measures have failed, the NPA can be considered, though caution should be exercised. Head injury is thus a **relative contraindication** to the use of an NPA.
The method of placement is to first size the diameter of the NPA directly against the size of the nasal opening. The correct size should allow the lubricated tip of the NPA to fit snuggly into the nose (**Fig. 1.5a**). The tip should be gently rotated in a twisting motion and aimed directly backward, not upward. If there is resistance to passing the NPA, do not force it: try the other nostril instead. If there is resistance using the other nostril, consider a smaller NPA.
The main complication of this airway is iatrogenic trauma resulting in blood passing into the player's airway from the nose (**Fig. 1.5b**).

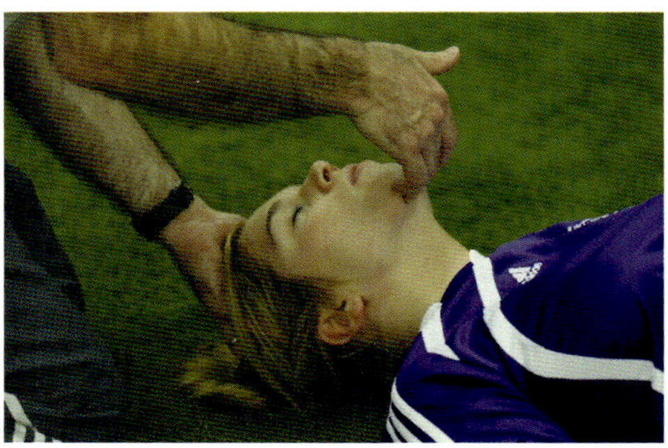

Fig. 1.3 Head tilt and chin lift.

Advanced Airway Adjuncts

While advanced airway adjuncts are very useful, it is far more important to do the basics well than to attempt a more advanced technique and fail due to lack of experience.

Laryngeal Mask Airway

The laryngeal mask airway (LMA) is an advanced airway tool that has found great use in the controlled environment of planned, fasted "routine" surgery. It is also a rescue airway tool used where there is a failure to intubate, as it is relatively quick and simple to use and provides a better degree of airway support than an NPA or Guedel.

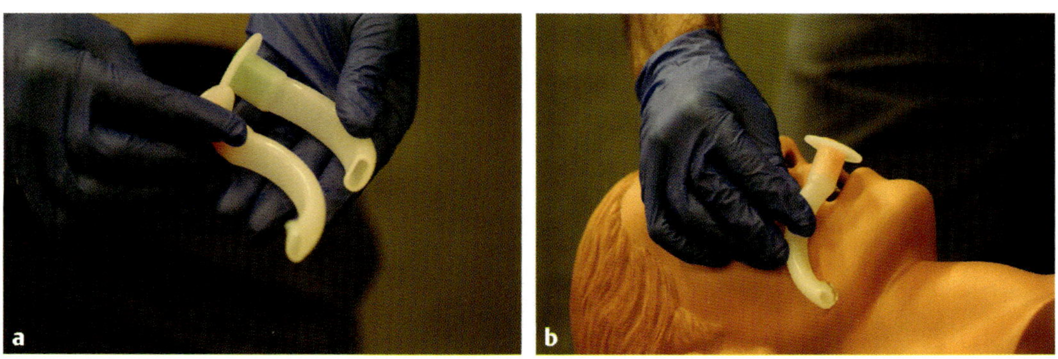

Fig. 1.4 **(a)** Guedel airway. **(b)** Sizing a Guedel airway.

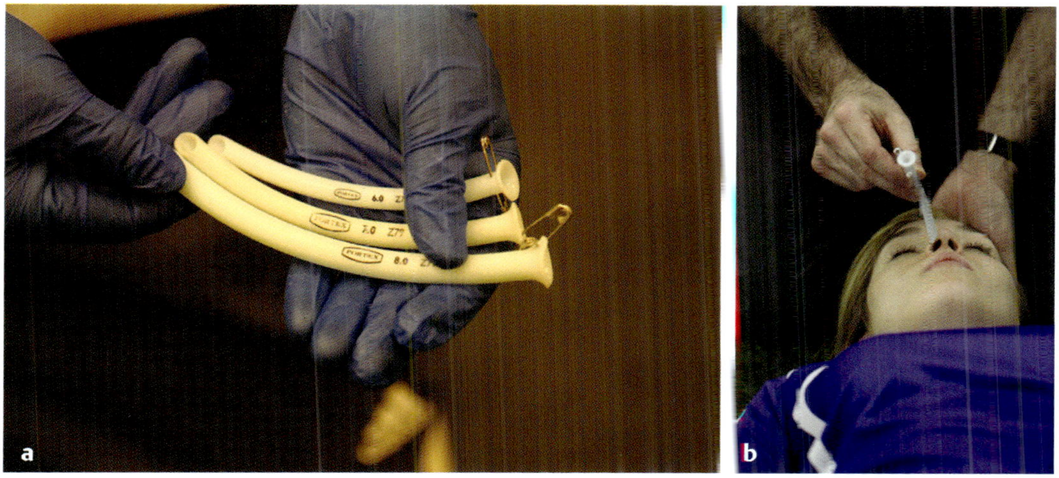

Fig. 1.5 (a) Nasopharyngeal airway. (b) Demonstration.

As with all other airway adjuncts, it comes in a range of sizes. On average, a size 4 or 5 is about right for a man and a size 4 for a woman.

An LMA is basically a plastic tube attached to a moldable, conforming inflatable end piece that should sit in the laryngopharynx when inflated.

When the LMA pack is opened, the moldable end piece should be placed on a flat surface and any remaining air removed using a syringe so that it becomes flat. It is then placed directly into the mouth and as far into the laryngopharynx as possible.

Once inflated, the whole airway will rise up a little if it is placed correctly. The player can then be bagged and an oxygen supply attached. There is better protection from secretions than found with an NPA or Guedel, but if the player vomits, then there is still a significant risk of aspiration, which is why an LMA must not be thought of as a definitive airway. The newer i-gel LMA come with a firm gel end piece that does not require inflation and as such is easier to use (see **Fig. 1.6**). Because it is preshaped to conform to airway anatomy, it is much less likely to be sited incorrectly. The only potential downside with the i-gel airways is that in extreme cold conditions the gel can start to freeze, making placement of the airway potentially much more difficult.

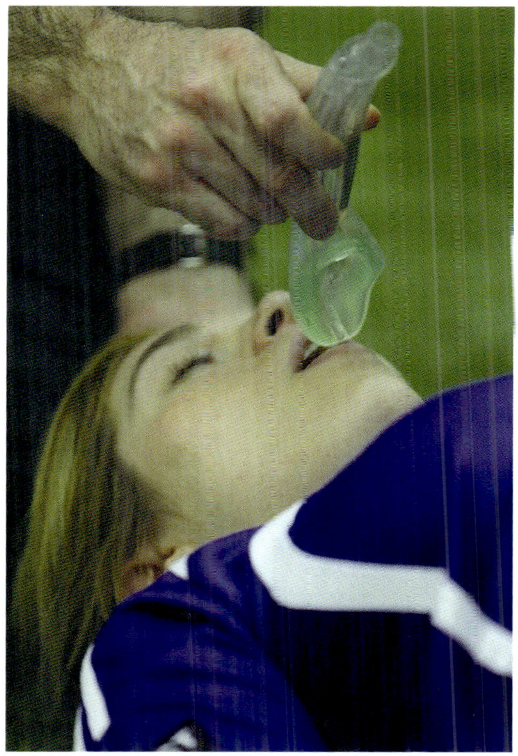

Fig. 1.6 Laryngeal mask airway.

Endotracheal Intubation

Intubation is considered the "gold standard" in airway management, but it is recommended that unless you practice intubation regularly, there is little benefit to you or the player in attempting to perform this technique.

Surgical Airways

Note: Surgical techniques have only been mentioned to allow a familiarity *in principle*. The methods for performing these are not included and specific training should be undertaken if you intend to perform such techniques.

Needle Cricothyroidotomy

A needle cricothyroidotomy is performed only when there is a proximal airway obstruction resulting in air being unable to flow into the

trachea despite all other adjuncts having been attempted. This is incredibly rare because the simple measures previously described will usually result in a player being able to be ventilated. A needle cricothyroidotomy may, however, be required due to significant facial trauma or anaphylaxis.
In order to be successful with a needle cricothyroidotomy, it is important that you have equipment with you that can be used to blow air into the trachea (e.g., an oxygen supply and connective tubing). This allows jet insufflation of oxygen into the lungs. Note that this will allow you to *oxygenate*, though not actually *ventilate* the player. A needle cricothyroidotomy should not be performed without this equipment as it will not achieve anything.
A needle cricothyroidotomy will give you around 30 minutes or so before the levels of carbon dioxide build up in the body, producing a fatal respiratory acidosis. For this reason, a needle cricothyroidotomy is very much a temporizing procedure to be followed by a formal surgical airway that will allow definitive airway control.
This technique should only be carried out if:

- **The player has a definite and complete proximal airway obstruction that is unresponsive to all basic interventions described above.**
- **The ambulance is delayed or no ambulance is available.**
- **You have access to a large caliber venflon, oxygen tubing, and an oxygen supply.**

Lastly, it must be re-emphasized that this procedure is only performed as a last-ditch effort to oxygenate a player in a highly unusual and uncommon clinical context.

Formal Surgical Airway

Along with endotracheal intubation of the trachea, a formal surgical airway is the only other method of formally "securing" the airway. As mentioned above, the needle cricothyroidotomy is a temporizing measure used when all other methods have failed and there is no one with the expertise to perform a formal surgical airway.
The formal surgical airway involves locating the cricothyroid membrane and cutting through this to allow the passage of a specific small-width tube that can be inflated to provide a seal across the trachea.
This type of procedure may be carried out using local anesthetic on an awake patient who is in the process of losing their airway due to burns, trauma, anaphylaxis, etc.

> **NOTE**
>
> To summarize, it is vital that you only practice techniques you are familiar with and do not feel pressured to perform advanced techniques when basic maneuvers would be more practical and useful.

1.3 The Cervical Spine

This should be immobilized by gently holding either side of the head in a neutral position (i.e., neither flexed nor extended) until the airway has been assessed. Assuming there is no issue with the airway, an assessment of the neck can then be made.
As mentioned above, the level of concern about a neck injury is directly related to the severity of the mechanism by which the injury was sustained. A number of guidelines have been drawn up that suggest that the cervical spine can be considered "cleared" if **all of the following** have been achieved:

- **Absence of posterior midline cervical spine tenderness.**
- **GCS of 15.**
- **Absence of focal neurological deficit—on motor or sensory testing.**
- **Absence of any distracting injuries.**
- **Ability to achieve active 45-degree lateral neck rotation in both directions.**
- **No concern over the mechanism of injury.**

Note: A distracting injury is one deemed significant enough by the assessing clinician to cause so much pain as to distract the player from the possibility of recognizing that they also have a cervical spine injury (i.e., long bone fracture, visceral injury, etc.).
If all of the above criteria are met then the neck can be "cleared" and hands removed from the head. If any of the above criteria are not met, then the cervical spine should be immobilized fully using an appropriately sized hard (also known as a semirigid) cervical collar and a spinal board, with blocks applied to each side of the head and taped. The player should only be moved on and off the spinal board by log roll with sufficient people to assist.
An alternative method to using a spinal board is a scoop stretcher and/or a vacuum mattress. These are perfectly valid methods of transporting an injured athlete with a potential neck injury as long as an appropriately sized and applied hard collar is in place, with blocks and tape.
Remember, the cervical spine is considered immobilized when either of the following is the case:

- The player has been placed on a spinal board (or scoop stretcher or vacuum mattress), a hard collar has been applied and the forehead taped onto the spinal board by placing tape from one side of the board to the other across the forehead and over the chin. Sandbags or blocks are then applied on either side of the head to complete the immobilization.
- Your hands are placed either side of the head to stop movement (with or without a hard collar on).

The neck is **not considered fully immobilized if the player only has a hard collar** on.

The drawback of option 2 is that it takes one person to hold the neck at all times. The benefit is that the clinician can maintain a jaw thrust at the same time—usually much easier if the hard collar is not on.

See Sections 4.1.4 and 4.1.5 in Chapter 4 of this volume for details on how to apply a hard collar and how to perform a log roll.

The player is unconscious and lying on their side.

In this situation, a log roll is required to move the player in a supported manner into a supine position (lying on their back). This usually requires three people—one each to take control of the thorax, the pelvis, and the lower limbs. The person holding the head has control of the maneuver and the player is gently turned on the command of this person.

The player is unconscious and vomiting. How do I protect the neck?

This is a potentially dangerous situation for someone who does not have a protected airway and is thus at serious risk of aspiration. While the temptation is to turn the head to the side or to move the player into the recovery position this would pose a significant risk to the spine as well. The solution is again to perform a log roll so that the player is rolled onto one side (opposite to that of any associated injury). This will allow any vomit to drain out of the side of the mouth. This maneuver can also be performed with the patient on a spinal board.

The player is combative and confused. Will restraining the neck make things worse?

In this situation, there is a risk of creating a fulcrum from fixing the head while the body is allowed to move freely. This can create forces that twist or flex the cervical spine and can result in the worsening of any existing injury.

A decision has to be made about what will cause most risk and potential harm to the player. Most injured players can be talked to, calmed down, and reassured, which will allow you to keep the spine immobilized.

If the player is thrashing about, then the best option is to remove the tape across the forehead and chin, but maintain the hard collar if possible. As stated above, you now have a situation with a player who has only a partly restrained spine, but this is still preferable to converting a stable spine injury into an unstable one.

The best advice is to *immediately transfer* the player by ambulance while maintaining a cervical collar if at all possible wherever there is any ongoing risk to the airway or spine.

1.4 Breathing

The assessment of the respiratory system is purely based on identifying injuries that may have life-threatening consequences.

The assessment follows on directly from the assessment and management of the airway and cervical spine.

As part of the airway assessment and management, we are already aware that observation of chest movement helps to confirm whether a player is breathing or not. It is now important to assess chest movement more closely to ascertain the following:

- ✓ Respiratory rate.
- ✓ Respiratory effort.
- ✓ Symmetry of chest movement
  - Look for an obvious lack of movement on one side of the chest.
  - Look for an obvious flail segment caused by fractures of three or more ribs and in two or more places in each of the affected ribs (this results in paradoxical breathing where the flail segment is pulled inward on inspiration and outward on exhalation).

Listen to the player both in terms of what they are saying and the respiratory noises they are making.

Gurgling implies upper airway pathology.
Stridor implies upper airway pathology.
Coughing is a protective reflex and a positive sound.
Wheezing implies lower respiratory tract pathology.

1

- Check trachea is central.
- Feel the neck for surgical emphysema.
- Feel the chest wall to assess pain or crepitus suggestive of a rib fracture.

It is unlikely that using a stethoscope will add anything to the initial pitchside assessment. If you suspect a pneumothorax is a possibility, then remove the player immediately and continue the assessment in the treatment room.

1.4.1 Practical Airway and Breathing Management

The player is not breathing.
Immediately check for a pulse. If there is no pulse, then immediately call for help and proceed with cardiopulmonary resuscitation (CPR; see Chapter 2 of this volume).

The player has a pulse but is not breathing properly.
Attempt a jaw thrust in the first instance, proceeding to an airway adjunct if the jaw thrust is not helping.

The player is still not breathing despite airway-opening maneuvers but does have a pulse.
This is a highly unusual situation on a field of play and would most likely occur secondary to another problem, such as obtundation caused by cerebral depression, either from trauma or iatrogenically after a benzodiazepine administered for seizure activity. Assisted ventilations are required at this point. These can either be basic or advanced.

- *Basic*—Use an airway-opening maneuver with an airway adjunct as described above, with a bag valve mask (BVM) attached to oxygen.
- *Advanced* —Intubation is the only way to truly secure the airway.

The player is in pain, is struggling to breathe, and has a clinical rib fracture.
In this situation, the management depends entirely on the rest of the assessment you make. As a minimum, the player needs a full assessment of pulse and BP, as well as a respiratory examination comprising air entry, chest percussion, tracheal deviation, and O_2 saturations where available. If all of these parameters are normal, then provide analgesia and reassess.
If there is decreased air entry, then the suspicion of a pneumothorax is raised and transfer to hospital is a sensible next step. **Do not give nitrous oxide as analgesia to anyone you suspect has a broken rib or pneumothorax** as this will preferentially diffuse into the pleural space, thus worsening any pneumothorax present.

The player is in pain, is struggling to breathe, and has a clinical pneumothorax.
Here you should check the vital signs as a matter of urgency, particularly to ensure that the player does not have a tension pneumothorax. This is a pneumothorax resulting in **associated shock** due to impaired venous return to the heart because the pneumothorax has become so large as to cause compression of the mediastinal structures and thus venous return to the heart. See Chapter 4 in this volume for more details on management of a tension pneumothorax.
(Shock is defined as a failure to perfuse the vital organs and will manifest itself as lowered or unrecordable BP and usually an associated tachycardia, unless the player is in peri-arrest, in which case they may be bradycardic.)
If the vital signs are normal, then oxygenate the player, provide analgesia, and transfer to hospital.

The player has a flail segment.
A flail segment is an unusual complication of a chest injury in sport. The treatment here is to oxygenate, provide analgesia, and transfer to hospital, where a decision can be made as to whether or not a chest drain or supported ventilation is required. Should the vital signs deteriorate, consider the possibility of a tension pneumothorax associated with the injury.

The player has a sucking chest wound. What is this and how do I manage it?
This is exceptionally uncommon in sport as it is usually the result of penetrating trauma. The pathology is basically an open pneumothorax resulting from a wound to the chest wall that is so large (two-thirds the size of the trachea) that on each inspiration the chest cavity preferentially fills with air instead of air passing into the lungs. This is potentially life-threatening and requires oxygenation, analgesia, and an occlusive dressing to be taped over the wound at three edges, **leaving one corner free** to allow air to escape on exhalation.

1.5 Circulation

Assessment of the circulatory system involves an assessment of the vital organs to decide whether they are being perfused or not. A player can bleed internally or externally, and clearly internal bleeding will not be as visibly apparent as external bleeding, such as from a compound fracture or scalp wound. Again, the assessment comes back to basics.

What is the player's skin color?

Someone who is pale and sweaty in a sporting situation is most likely to be suffering from excessive vagal stimulation due to pain. This should be resolved very quickly just by lying them supine on the ground. If the player remains pale and with localizing pain to one area, then it is important to focus on assessment of this area. A kick to the left flank may result in an injury to either the spleen, kidney, or chest wall, for example.

Is there any visible deformity?

There is a great temptation to focus on the ankle pointing the wrong way, the dislocated shoulder, or the bleeding wound without first assessing airway and breathing. The aim here is to control further blood loss regardless of whether that bleeding is visible or invisible. Most wounds will stop bleeding when direct pressure is applied and a plentiful supply of gauze swabs is strongly advised. Any visible wound should have pressure applied while you quickly ascertain that there is no issue with the airway, the cervical spine, or breathing. Once this is done, you can focus on a circulatory assessment while bearing in mind the injury in front of you.

Listen to the player. What happened? What information can they tell you?

Pulse rate

In general terms, the maximum heart rate that should be expected of an athlete is 220 minus their age. So, if assessing a 38-year-old footballer, you should not expect to find a pulse of 200 beats per minute. If that is the case, the likely diagnosis is a supraventricular tachycardia (SVT) or possibly, though less likely, a ventricular tachycardia (VT).

Capillary refill time

This is a useful, if often overlooked, part of the clinical assessment. The capillary refill time (CRT) is measured by pressing your thumb on the player's sternum for a count of 5 seconds. Quickly release your thumb and count how long it takes for normal skin color to return to the area blanched by your thumb. This should take less than 2 seconds. If it does not, the suspicion of a serious clinical problem with either breathing or circulation is raised.

This assessment can be carried out anywhere and on anyone of any age. Do not be tempted to use peripheral capillary refill (e.g., a finger) for this purpose, as this will be much more liable to be affected by other factors such as cold weather.

Blood pressure

This is an assessment only carried out in the dressing room, treatment room, or ambulance. There is no indication to perform this at pitchside.

Should you feel the need to check a player's BP, then by definition they will not be returned to the field of play and thus should quickly be removed from it.

Measuring BP is a useful procedure when carried out in the appropriate setting. Like pulse and CRT, it is something that can be done serially, allowing a trend or pattern to become apparent.

To avoid false readings, make sure that the cuff you use is of an appropriate size for the player

Blood sugar

Any unconscious, confused, or fitting player should have their blood glucose checked as a matter of urgency, irrespective of whether or not they are known to be diabetic.

Administering glucagon or concentrated dextrose to a hypoglycemic player will quickly address these issues and will likely resolve the clinical situation. Being aware of athletes in your care who suffer from diabetes is essential preparation for managing these types of situation. Doctors should be aware that often many players may feel disinclined to share this information with the team clinician in case judgments are then made about their fitness to play. This may be the case even when they are in otherwise excellent health.

1.5.1 Assess Abdomen

A visual assessment should be made for signs of bruising or wounds. This is followed by palpation of the abdomen looking for guarding or peritonism. If there is ongoing alteration in vital signs as discussed above, the player should receive analgesia and be transferred to hospital for further assessment.

Splenic injuries in particular may take a few hours to become clinically apparent and if the mechanism is of concern, the diagnosis should not be dismissed even if the initial examination appears normal.

1.5.2 Assess Pelvis

Any downward or posterior movement could worsen a pelvic fracture by opening it outward. If an assessment of the stability of the pelvis needs to be made, it should involve firmly holding onto the iliac crests and pulling **inward**, never downward. Instead, compressing the pelvis inward, while potentially eliciting pain, is certainly unlikely to worsen it or cause harm. **This assessment should be made only once.**

1.5.3 Assess Long Bones

Fractures of the femur have the potential to bleed up to 1 to 1.5 L of blood if closed. In the event of a compound fracture, this blood loss can double. It is therefore clear that an assessment of the long bones of the lower limbs is essential as part of the circulation assessment. Reduction and splinting of any fracture should be performed as quickly as possible to minimize pain and bleeding.

The player has a bleeding scalp wound and appears pale and confused. Is concussion or blood loss causing the confusion?

Here, the first priority is again to go back to basics. Start at the airway while assuming a potential problem with the cervical spine.

The scalp wound may be a distracting injury not only for the player, but also for you as the clinician. Your responsibility is to make sure you apply the fundamentals of assessment and assess A and B fully before moving onto pulse, BP, etc.

Confusion due to blood loss is not likely in a player you have watched being injured from the touchlines, as the assessment you make will take place very soon after the injury is sustained.

In this case, the likelihood is that the player is concussed. However, there are other possibilities, such as a hypoglycemic player who sustained an injury because of a lack of awareness of their surroundings immediately beforehand. Either way, any player with a decreased GCS needs to be removed **safely** from the field of play so that a full assessment can be carried out to ascertain the cause of the problem.

While this may appear a basic and relatively straightforward problem to manage, you must still give due consideration to the potential pitfalls of the head injury such as cervical spine injury and other causes of confusion such as hypoxia from a pneumothorax. Likewise, a straightforward blood glucose may also give you the answer.

The player has sustained a direct blow to the shin and has a compound fracture. What are the next steps?

First, you must resist treating the fracture and take a few seconds to address and exclude any potentially life-threatening injuries that may have been sustained as part of the obvious injury. This should only take a few *seconds*. Your eyes will tell you most of what you need to know: with a long bone fracture, the player is unlikely to be rolling about on the pitch.

Take the time to ensure that you are not missing anything else about the injury. This will be time well spent while you compose yourself to deal with the issue of the fractured lower limb. Until you know the extent of the injury, you must assume the fracture is unstable and also assume it affects the joints both above and below the fracture site. Splinting these areas will allow you to move the player safely and effectively.

1.6 Disability

This is basically an assessment of the player's conscious level and also a neurological assessment (**Fig. 1.7**). It is vital for anyone with a suspected neck or head injury, and can be broken down into three main components:

- Conscious level.
- Pupils.
- Localizing (lateralizing) signs.

1.6.1 Conscious Level

There are two main scoring systems used to quickly assess the conscious level, and it is vital when treating emergency cases that you only use the one you are most familiar with. The AVPU scoring system is recommended over the GCS unless you are comfortable that you can assess the player by this latter system and **fully remember** its three different components.

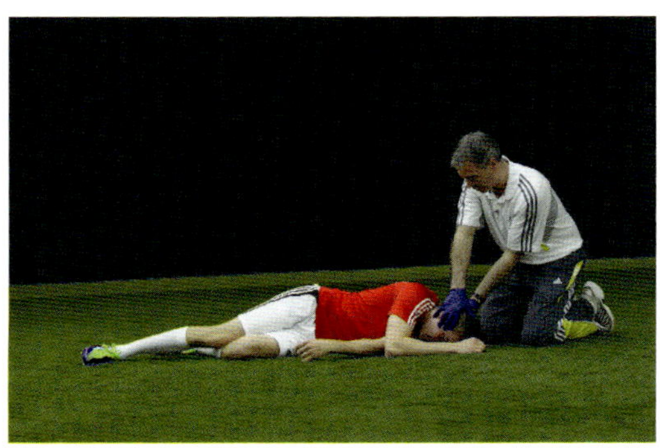

Fig. 1.7 Assessing a neck injury.

Table 1.1

The AVPU scoring system

			Equivalent GCS score
A	Alert	The player is fully conscious and responds appropriately.	15
V	Verbal	The player responds to verbal command as a stimulus.	13
P	Pain	The player responds to painful stimulus (see GCS regarding the stimulus).	8
U	Unresponsive	There is no response to painful stimulus.	3

Alert, Verbal, Pain, Unresponsive Scoring System

The AVPU scoring system is widely used as part of the initial assessment as it is reliable and easily repeated (**Table 1.1**). **Note:** You will see that the AVPU exactly mirrors the "eye" component of the GCS. When using the AVPU, anything less than an alert response mandates the removal of a player from the field of play, and a full assessment must be made.

Glasgow Coma Scale

The GCS is a validated scoring system in trauma and is a far more comprehensive but potentially more difficult assessment to make than the AVPU. The score is based on three components to give a total of between 3 and 15 (**Table 1.2**).

Method. If the player does not respond to verbal command, a painful stimulus should be carried out by the clinician by pinching the athlete's trapezius muscle on one side of the neck. It is important that you only attempt either a verbal **or** a painful stimulus at any one time, as doing both at exactly the same time will not help you differentiate which stimulus the player is actually responding to.

Anything less than a full GCS score of 15 mandates removal from the field of play.

Most neurosurgeons would consider the motor response as more important than either verbal or eye, and it is vital to make sure that you are absolutely clear which motor response you have elicited. As mentioned previously, the painful stimulus is applied using a trapezius pinch or squeeze.

- A **localizing** response will involve the player reaching his arm up to pull the clinician's fingers away to stop his neck being pinched. This movement toward the painful stimulus here should be a purposeful one and should reach **above the level of the clavicle.**

Table 1.2

Glasgow Coma Scale

Category	Response	Score[a]
Eyes[b]	Open spontaneously	4
	Open to verbal command	3
	Open to pain	2
	Do not open	1
Motor	Obeys commands	6
	Localizes to painful stimulus	5
	Withdraws from painful stimulus	4
	Flexes to painful stimulus	3
	Extends to painful stimulus	2
	No response to pain	1
Verbal	Orientated	5
	Confused	4
	Inappropriate	3
	Incomprehensible	2
	No verbal response	1

[a]*The score is **the best score** you elicit. So a player who is localizing on one side but not moving the other side at all would score 5 for his motor response. The lowest total score possible is 3, not 0.*
[b]*This part of the assessment mirrors the AVPU.*

- A **withdrawal** response will involve the player trying to pull away from the painful stimulus. In the case of the trapezius pinch, this will probably involve the player trying to turn their head away or possibly even their upper body a little as well. If you are unsure if this is definitely the response you are getting, then try a fingertip squeeze instead and the player will pull their hand away from you.
- A **flexion** (decorticate) response is best described as a bending of the upper limb, most visibly noticed at the elbow. This gives a similar type of movement as seen in the localizing response, but the arms are not flexing in a purposeful way and as such are unlikely to reach past the level of the clavicles as they are not trying to push away the stimulus. Here the lower limbs will extend in response to the painful stimulus.
- The **extension** (decerebrate) response involves both upper and lower limbs extending to pain, with the upper arms internally rotated too.

The distinction between localizing and flexing is probably the most difficult one and it is recommended you apply the trapezius squeeze and use the level of the clavicles as a cutoff point.

If in doubt about withdrawing, use a fingertip squeeze. Do not use the fingertip squeeze to decide between localizing and flexing.

1

1.6.2 Pupils

Both direct and consensual pupillary responses are a very useful aspect of the neurological exam. The most worrying finding in an unconscious player would be a fixed and dilated pupil suggesting compression of the oculomotor nerve due to increased intracranial pressure from a bleed. It is possible to find this in someone with a GCS of 15, but exceptionally rare. It is usually associated with other factors such as vomiting or headache.

You should bear in mind that a number of other diagnoses can be suggested from the varying appearances you may find. Examining the pupils early on allows a baseline from which to make serial assessments. This is important to allow you to recognize the various "incidental" appearances you may find. It is not unusual to find one pupil slightly larger than the other and this may be normal for the athlete. Other conditions such as Holmes–Adie syndrome may also cause confusion for the assessing clinician, so the physical condition of the player must be taken into consideration and clinical context applied.

Traumatic mydriasis is the result of a direct blow to the orbit. It may be present in isolation or may indicate a blowout fracture or even a bleed into the anterior chamber of the eye if associated with a hyphema.

Bilateral pinpoint pupils may suggest an opiate ingestion—not likely in a professional setting, but a possible cause of collapse in the amateur game or a reflection of a player taking nonprescription medications for an ongoing injury. Likewise, bilateral dilated pupils may represent ingestion of amphetamine, tricyclics, or even local instillation of eye drops. It will also be found in any player who has received atropine or adrenaline and should never be used in isolation as a clinical endpoint on which to end a resuscitation.

NOTE

If a player has a head trauma, a decreased GCS, and one fixed, dilated pupil, the cause of this will be an intracranial bleed on the ipsilateral (same) side as the dilated pupil. This condition necessitates immediate neurosurgical decompression.

1.6.3 Localizing Signs

This is basically a rapid assessment to try to "localize" any neurological problem (either brain or spinal cord) that is clearly resulting in a neurological deficit. It is a gross assessment of motor and sensory function.

If the player is GCS 15, then asking about weakness, numbness, or tingling is a useful starting point. This should progress onto a physical assessment of the tone and power of upper limbs, assessing both sides at the same time to look for a discrepancy. The same should then be carried out on the lower limbs too.

In the vast majority of cases, most players with a GCS of 15 will readily demonstrate normal gross neurology once their cervical spine has been cleared. If there is a concern about a player's history or symptoms, remove them from the field of play and perform a full neurological assessment.

Chapter 2

Cardiac Arrest and Choking

Jonny Gordon

2.1 Cardiac Arrest

2

The European Resuscitation Council (ERC) Guidelines 2015 emphasize the importance of providing effective cardiopulmonary resuscitation (CPR) and early defibrillation where possible. The guidelines stipulate that chest compressions should be as uninterrupted as possible. The ratio of compressions to ventilations is 30:2.

Depth of compression should be 5 to 6 cm with the rate of compression 100 to 120 per minute.

Once CPR has started, it should not stop unless the victim shows signs of life such as a return to consciousness **in addition** to a return to normal breathing.

The basic life support algorithm acknowledges that many inexperienced or laypersons may struggle to identify someone in cardiac arrest. As a result of this, the ERC suggests starting chest compressions in anyone who is both unresponsive and not breathing normally. This is helpful for those with absolutely no experience to fall back on, but it is the aim of this manual and the course to encourage those who have had some experience in life support (however rusty) to apply a more advanced approach even to the basic life support algorithm.

2.1.1 Adult Basic Life Support

Outside the confines of a hospital or general practice surgery where there is no access to cardiac monitors, defibrillators, etc., it can be challenging even to ascertain that the patient has in fact suffered a cardiac arrest.

The ability to palpate and accurately comment on the presence or absence of a pulse in a cardiac arrest has been shown to be more technically difficult than was previously thought. Also, in the immediate phase after cardiac output has failed, the patient may appear to be suffering from a seizure when in actual fact the seizure is the result of cerebral hypoxia caused by failure to perfuse the cerebrum. These factors together can make the diagnosis of a cardiac arrest more difficult and the limitations in assessment that each causes should be borne in mind.

NOTE

Remember, basic life support is only basic in terms of the level of kit necessary to carry it out.

If you have access to more advanced kit such as an airway adjunct or a defibrillator, you should ensure you are familiar with its use wherever possible (**Fig. 2.1**). Dealing with an arrest is not the best time to start familiarizing yourself with the equipment at your disposal.

Assess Responsiveness

- Whilst the algorithm has been simplified in terms of the number of steps presented, the assessments of airway and breathing are still included practically.
- Once unresponsiveness has been ascertained, make an assessment as to whether the player is breathing or not. This will involve an airway assessment and opening of the airway with a jaw thrust (or possibly head tilt and chin lift if there is no concern regarding the cervical spine).
- Look listen and feel as described in the initial assessment for signs of breathing.
- Feel for a pulse at the same time and look for signs of life, i.e. is the player moving, groaning etc.
- If there is a problem with either the player not breathing or with the brief circulation assessment you have just made (no pulse or signs of life), then **immediately call for an ambulance** and start 30 chest compressions (**Fig. 2.2**).

Should you been unfortunate enough to find yourself alone at this point, and with no access to a mobile phone to call for help you must leave the casualty and get help *before* starting any other treatments. This is vital because defibrillation is the cornerstone of treatment in the 'shockable' rhythms and this cannot be done unless you have a defibrillator with you.

Chest Compressions

- *Location* of compressions: hands directly over the middle of the chest.
- *Depth* of compressions: **5 to 6 cm.**
- *Rate* of compressions: **100 to 120 bpm.**

It is likely that you may perform the compressions much faster than this, but the faster the rate, the less time there is for the coronary arteries to be perfused on the upstroke of the compression (diastole).

Once you have completed your 30 compressions, immediately perform two ventilations. Then continue compressions and ventilations at a ratio of 30:2.

2.1.2 Automated External Defibrillation

Good-quality uninterrupted chest compressions and early defibrillation are the evidence-based treatments for anyone in cardiac arrest with a shockable rhythm.

The ability to cardiovert someone back to sinus rhythm with a pulse and signs of life is clearly related to how quickly they can be defibrillated. With every passing minute, the chances of a

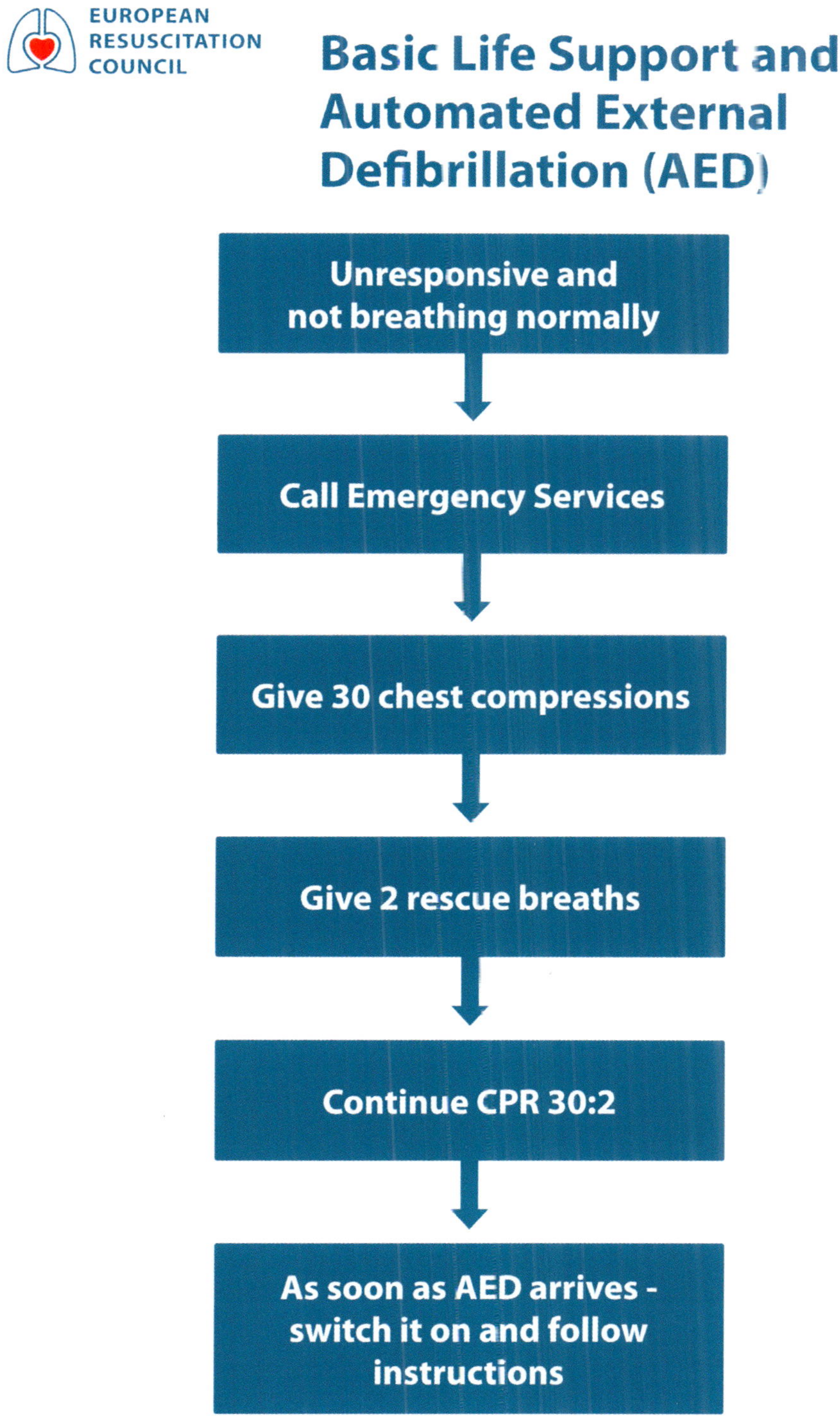

Fig. 2.1 Adult basic life support. (Copyright European Resuscitation Council – www.erc.edu – 2016_NGL_043)

successful defibrillation decrease by up to 10%. The automated external defibrillator (AED) is a device that can be used quickly and easily, and is far more readily available and accessible now than ever before. **Make sure your AED is programmed with the 2015 guidelines**—you should check with your manufacturer to ensure this is the case and update if necessary.

If an AED is part of the kit you take with you to look after a team, make sure you have ready access to it and are familiar with how it works. It will be of no use in the medical hamper at the hotel if you have to manage a cardiac event during training.

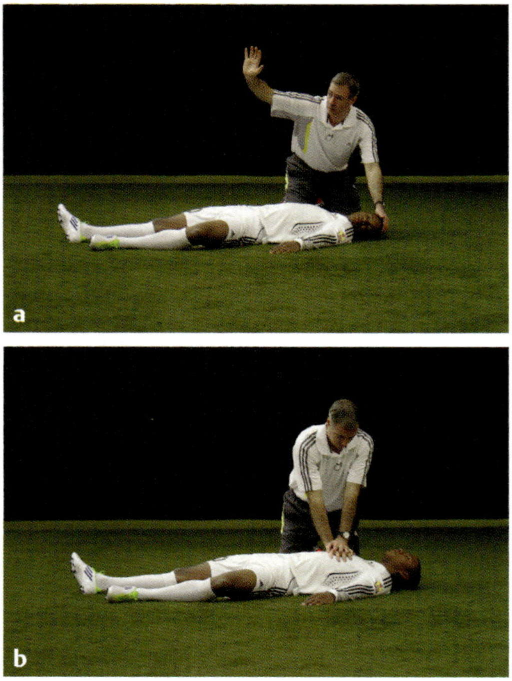

Fig. 2.2 Immediately call for help **(a)**, then start chest compressions **(b)**.

The kit will prompt you at all stages. It is designed to be used by a layperson and should also be relatively familiar to those who use manual defibrillators in their day-to-day clinical practice. You will be guided both by verbal commands from the machine and by visual stimulus with the adhesive pads showing the placement. One pad should be placed to the right of the sternum under the clavicle and the second to the left lateral chest wall just below the left nipple (**Fig. 2.3**).

Some types of machine are fully automatic and require no input other than attachment of the pads; others are semiautomatic, with the potential for an override function to be used by an experienced clinician.

The two main considerations when using an AED are the following:

- To recognize that the player requires it in the first place (any unresponsive collapse).
- To ensure the safety of everyone who is assisting you.

Post-2003, most machines are now biphasic, delivering shocks in the region of 200 J once the internal capacitor has charged.

An AED may be safely used on a child over the age of 8 years. On patients between the ages of 1 and 8 years, pediatric pads should be used to attenuate the electrical charge, but if no pediatric pads are available, use the adult pads. When treating under-1-year-olds with no pediatric pads available, there is no consensus as to whether to use the adult pads alone though the advice is to consider doing so (**Fig. 2.4**).

2.1.3 Airway Management in Cardiac Arrest

As discussed earlier, if your assessment of the player reveals someone who is unresponsive, an immediate airway assessment is necessary to ascertain whether they are breathing. This should incorporate airway-opening maneuvers. **Remember: if you find the**

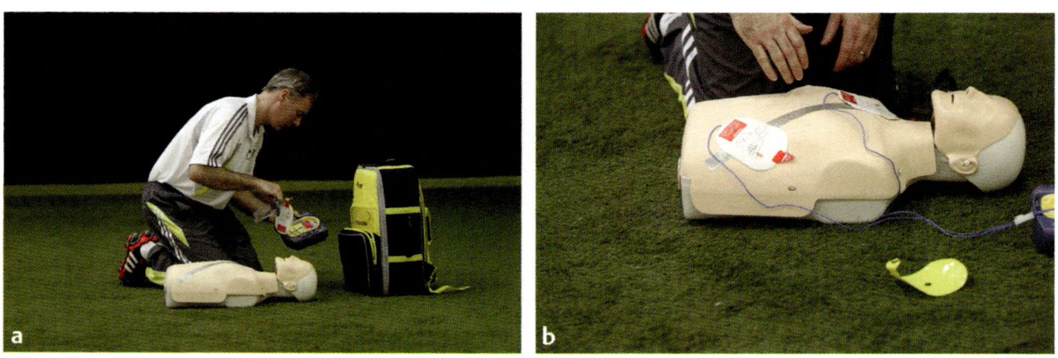

Fig. 2.3 Preparing **(a)** and fitting a defibrillator **(b)**.

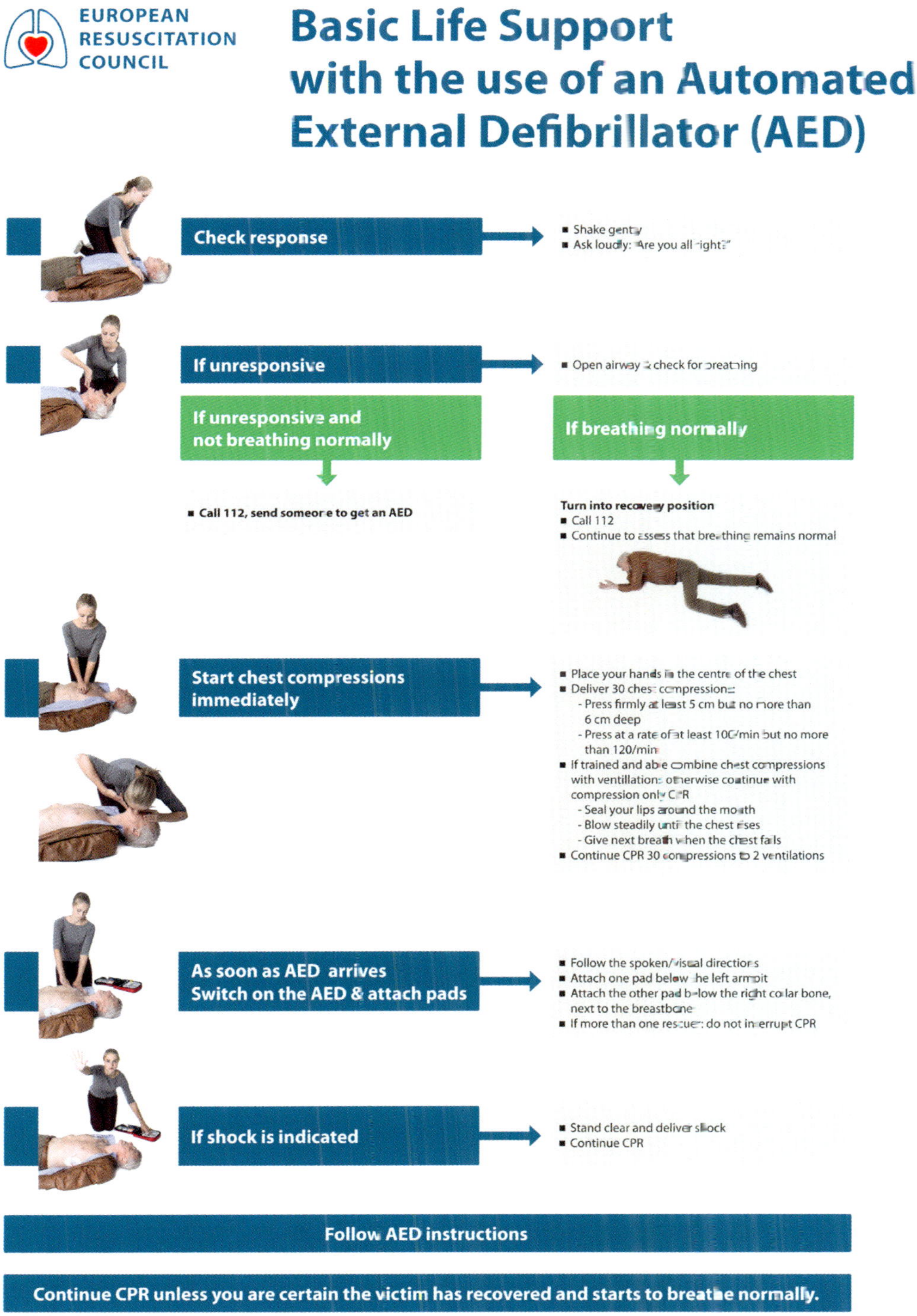

Fig. 2.4 Automated external defibrillation. (Copyright European Resuscitation Council – www.erc.edu – 2016_NGL_043.)

player is not breathing, the next step is to attach the AED if available, rather than securing the airway.

When it comes to managing the airway, the same techniques as described in Chapter 1 apply here, although there are other advanced skills that may be applicable too, depending on your level of experience.

Management of the airway can be divided into four sections as described in Chapter 1 of this volume:

- Airway-opening maneuvers.
- Basic airway adjuncts.
- Advanced airway adjuncts.
- Surgical airways.

Whatever combination of techniques you use, it is vital that you ALWAYS use the maximum amount of oxygen available to you and NEVER try to carry out an advanced skill that you are not trained to perform.

NOTE

You are more likely to succeed in resuscitating someone by doing the simple things very well.

The reason for including these more advanced techniques is not to teach them to you or for you to think that you should be performing them, but to allow you to be clear in your mind what each one is and when it may be appropriate—in the right hands—for them to be carried out.

2.1.4 Potentially Reversible Causes of Cardiac Arrest

The immediate management of cardiac arrest is focused on providing well-performed chest compressions and airway support along with immediate defibrillation where applicable. It is also important to try to identify and treat any potentially reversible causes of the cardiac arrest.

These are best divided into eight groups of potentially reversible causes: the four Hs and the four Ts (**Table 2.1**).

Clearly in the setting of the sports arena most of these are unlikely to occur, and in any case would perhaps be undiagnosable with limited equipment. Focus must be placed on assessing the assessable and treating the treatable—namely, hypoxia, hypovolaemia, tension pneumothorax and possibly hypothermia (depending on the environment).

Remember to use the maximum concentration of oxygen available to you. Exhaled air has a concentration of approximately 15 to 17%. Airway management is as described earlier.

Hypovolemia progressing to cardiac arrest is most commonly due to blood loss. In the sporting context, an athlete suffering trauma resulting in cardiac arrest due to hypovolemia is unlikely to bleed out in the initial few minutes of assessment. Penetrating trauma accounts for most of these cases. In the context of blunt trauma, bleeding into any of the major body cavities, i.e., pleural, retroperitoneal, or intraperitoneal spaces, may even take hours to manifest itself clinically, and repeated observations of any athlete may be required to ensure the clinical situation is stable and nonchanging. It is unlikely in sport that hypovolemia would become such an issue as to progress to cardiac arrest without something else also needing to be addressed, such as electrolyte status or heat stroke.

Tension pneumothorax is a life-threatening condition that develops when a pneumothorax develops in size to the point that it causes compression of mediastinal structures and thus inhibits venous return to the heart, causing cardiac arrest. This occurs due to a valve effect that results in air being forced into the pleural space on inspiration, but this air cannot leave the space on expiration. It is uncommon but should be suspected in anyone who has sustained an injury to the chest and becomes increasingly short of breath. The doctor's job is to ensure the player does not deteriorate to the point of cardiac arrest before intervention takes place.

Poor air entry may be identified by looking at chest wall movement but should be readily confirmed on auscultation. Classic findings include tracheal deviation *away* from the side of the chest, the pneumothorax is on, and hyperresonance to chest wall percussion are unfortunately not always present. A tachycardia is inevitable and hypotension suggests impending circulatory collapse.

Treatment for this is to administer oxygen immediately at the maximum concentration available and to decompress the pressure in the pleural cavity. This is achieved by placing a cannula into the pleural space in the second intercostal space in the midclavicular line, thus allowing air to leave the pleural space. A formal chest drain should still be inserted, but once the cannula has decompressed the pleural space some time has been bought prior to a drain being necessary.

2.1.5 Advanced Adult Life Support

The adult algorithm quickly requires you to assess the cardiac rhythm and immediately treat any

Table 2.1

The four Hs and four Ts

Four Hs	Four Ts
Hypoxia	Tension pneumothorax
Hypovolemia	Tamponade (cardiac)
Hypothermia	Toxins
Hypokalemia/hyperkalemia	Thromboembolic (pulmonary)

shockable rhythm with defibrillation. A defibrillator is required for both assessment and treatment. If you do not have one, then it becomes even more important to call an ambulance. In the meantime, it is vital that you continue to perform basic life support as well as you possibly can, using cardiac compressions and supported airway ventilations at a ratio of 30:2.

Irrespective of the cause of a cardiac arrest, the treatment will be altered depending on the nature of the underlying rhythm, which is either shockable or nonshockable.

Shockable Rhythms

Ventricular Fibrillation. Ventricular fibrillation (VF) results in a chaotic baseline of electrical activity that does not generate any purposeful cardiac contraction and therefore does not generate any cardiac output (**Fig. 2.5**). If recognized on a monitor, it can be readily treated by defibrillation.

Pulseless Ventricular Tachycardia. Pulseless ventricular tachycardia (VT) is a broad complex tachycardia of ventricular origin that produces electrical complexes on the monitor but no meaningful cardiac output (**Fig. 2.6**). If a patient is on a monitor with a broad complex tachycardia and shows no signs of life, immediate defibrillation is again the treatment of choice, as with VF.

Nonshockable Rhythms

These rhythms are associated with a much poorer prognosis than VF or pulseless VT. CPR is the mainstay of treatment and it is vital to ensure this is carried out as well as possible. If oxygen is available, this should be used to maximal effect. If the patient is intubated, then ventilate using O_2; if ventilating using a pocket mask, then ensure the oxygen tubing fits in under the mask.

Asystole. The appearance in asystole is of a flatline trace (**Fig. 2.7**). You must check that the leads are on correctly and the gain is turned up (if applicable).

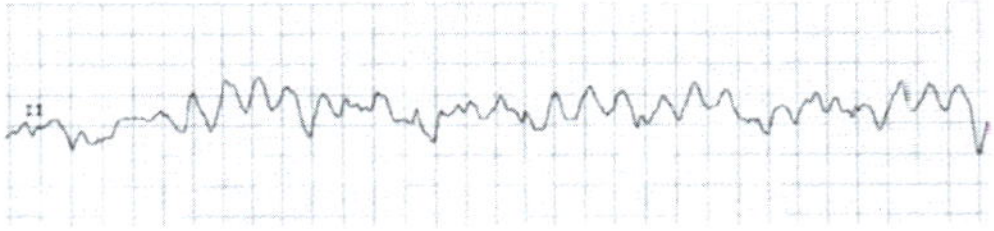

Fig. 2.5 Ventricular fibrillation – Chaotic baseline of electrical activity (electrocardiogram).

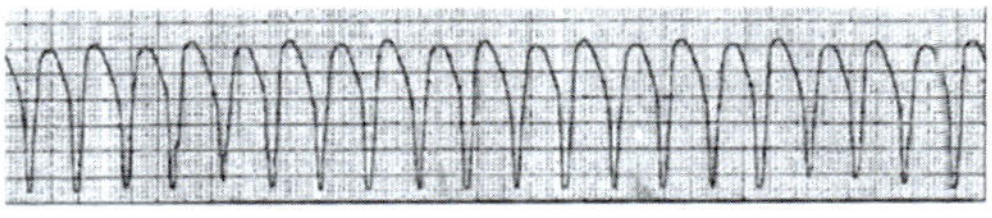

Fig. 2.6 Ventricular tachycardia – Broad complex tachycardia (electrocardiogram).

Pulseless Electrical Activity. In pulseless electrical activity (PEA; previously known as electromechanical dissociation [EMD]), electrical complexes are present on the monitor, but the cardiac output is either nonexistent or so limited as to prevent a discernible blood pressure from being generated. This causes failure to perfuse the brain, heart, and vital organs, and leads to a nonpalpable pulse.

Management of Shockable Rhythms

Once cardiac arrest has been confirmed and a shockable rhythm identified, immediate defibrillation is the first step. **Immediately after the shock is given, restart CPR** (30:2) without a pulse check or even checking the monitor and continue for a further 2 minutes or until the player shows signs of life (**Fig. 2.8**).

Note: Only one shock is given per cycle.

After the initial shock has been given (or diagnosis of shockable rhythm), the next shock and subsequent shocks are delivered at the end of every 2-minute cycle that passes. This equates to roughly five cycles of 30:2.

There appears to be no hard evidence regarding the energy for each shock. It is suggested this is initially 150 J for a biphasic, then anywhere between 150 and 360 J for each subsequent shock delivered. If using a monophasic, then every shock is given at 360 J. The monitor should be *quickly* checked after each 2 minutes of CPR. If this demonstrates a change to a nonshockable rhythm with evidence of organized complexes, carry out a pulse check.

Do not stop chest compressions if you see the rhythm change on the monitor during your 2-minute cycle **unless** the patient shows signs of life and starts to breathe normally.

Adrenaline (epinephrine) is no longer given immediately once a shockable rhythm and cardiac arrest have been identified. Instead, **adrenaline is given immediately after the third shock** at the start of the third cycle of 2 minutes, i.e., approximately 4 minutes after you first shock the patient. The dose is 1 mg intravenously. (Amiodarone 300 mg IV can be given at the same time.)

Adrenaline should be re-administered every 3 to 5 minutes, i.e., after every two cycles of 2 minutes of CPR.

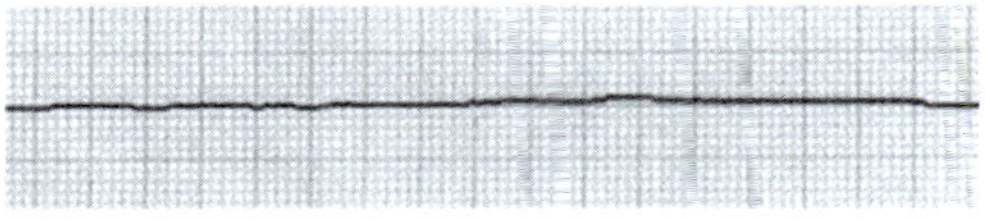

Fig. 2.7 Asystole–Flatline trace (electrocardiogram).

2

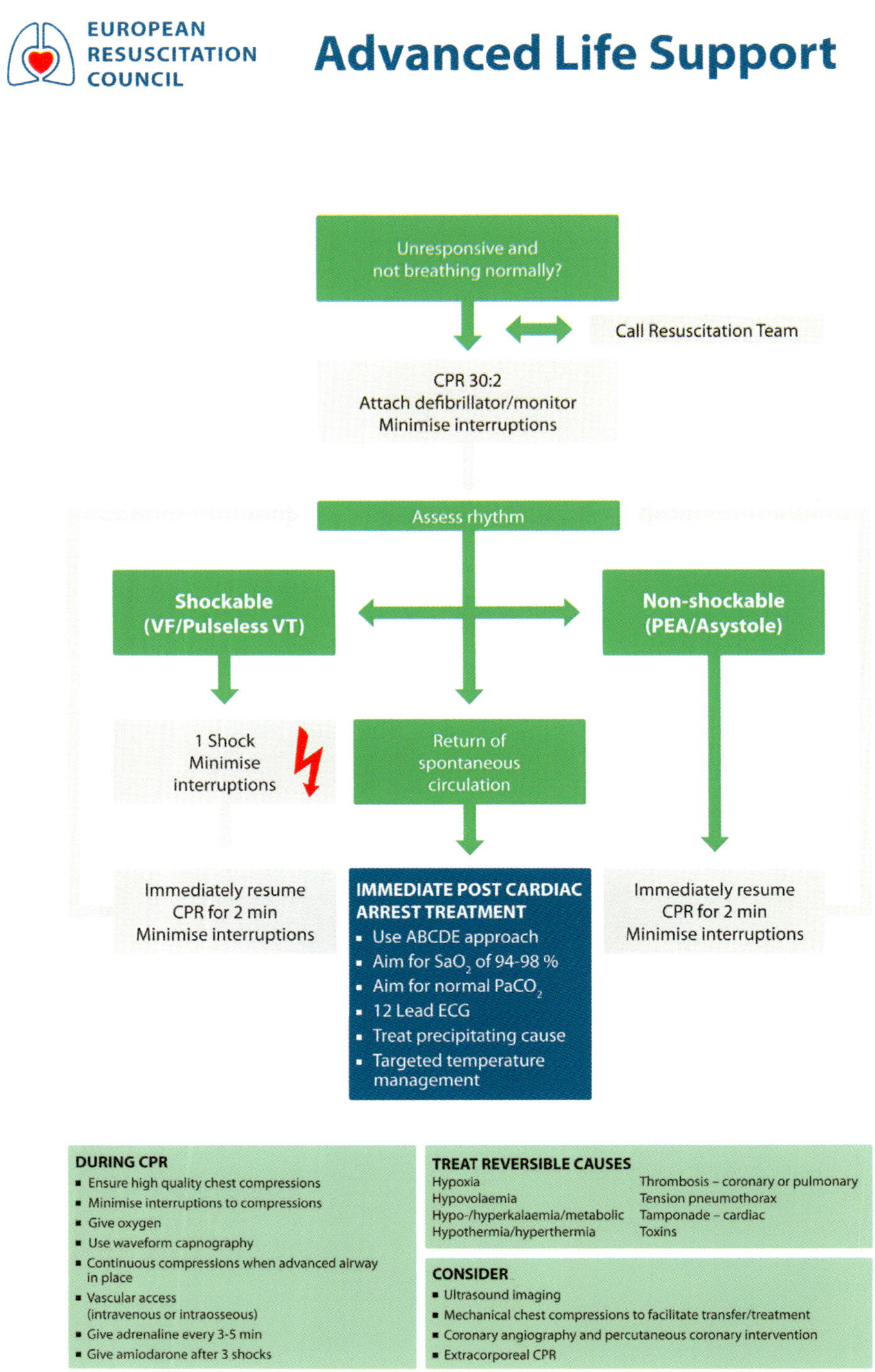

Fig. 2.8 Advanced life support. (Copyright European Resuscitation Council – www.erc.edu – 2016_NGL_043.)

Precordial Thump

The precordial thump is a technique recommended for any doctor who is treating a patient who has a *witnessed and monitored* collapse where a defibrillator is not immediately available. It is unlikely that you will find yourself with a player who fulfills these criteria in an out-of-hospital environment. This technique is most likely to be successful in converting pulseless VT. Limited success has been described with this technique in patients who are in VF, and when successful it has been carried out less than 10 seconds after the arrest. The role of the precordial thump was de-emphasized in the ERC 2010 guidelines unless the criteria previously mentioned are met.

The precordial thump is carried out by clenching your fist and dropping this from a height of about 20 cm (approximately the height of a football) directly onto the player's lower sternum. Immediately retract your hand to create an impulse-like stimulus. After performing this technique, check for a pulse. If no pulse is present, start CPR, get help if you have not done so already, and obtain a monitor or defibrillator if possible to assess rhythm.

Management of Nonshockable Rhythms

If you find a flatline trace on the monitor or defibrillator, ensure that the leads are attached correctly as the same appearance will be found with a disconnected lead.

The nonshockable algorithm differs from VF in that adrenaline 1 mg IV is given **immediately** once it is identified.

Atropine is no longer recommended by the ERC in either asystole or PEA.

If a patient who is initially in VF or pulseless VT is shocked into asystole, the next dose of adrenaline should be given approximately 3 to 5 minutes after the last dose. This reflects the half-life of adrenaline.

A further 2010 guideline change is that should IV access prove impossible, it is no longer recommended to **give adrenaline down an endotracheal tube.**

Basic or Advanced Life Support in Pitchside Cardiac Arrest?

It is vital to perform the basic assessments and treatment well, asking for help immediately, and then focusing on good effective CPR and use of the AED. In a pitchside cardiac arrest where an AED is present (and it is each clinician's responsibility to ensure this is the case), it is unlikely that the defibrillator will be of a type to show the rhythm.

Obviously if the machine recommends a shock, then it is completely appropriate to continue as you would down the "shockable" side of the algorithm and use the drugs administered intravenously (adrenaline and amiodarone) just after the third shock. Again, if no shock is advised, then give adrenaline immediately after you gain IV access, and treat down this side of the algorithm.

NOTE

Keep it structured, know your equipment, and know your team's abilities and limitations. You are more likely to succeed in resuscitating someone by doing the simple things very well.

2.2 Choking

It is vitally important to ascertain in anyone who is choking what has actually precipitated the incident. Any player may present to you where there is a clear history of choking on a foreign body, but this should be clearly distinguished from someone who presents to you with an upper airway obstruction without any obvious cause. In this situation, it is vital to consider the other possible causes, such as anaphylaxis or infection. The history will usually confirm the cause and there will usually be a history of recent eating. The person may be drooling, stridorous, coughing, or even apneic.

The algorithm shown in **Fig. 2.9** demonstrates the interventions required.

The main questions to consider are as follows:

- Can the person cough adequately?
- If they cannot cough adequately, are they conscious?

In mild airway obstruction, the player will cough adequately. Leave them in the most comfortable position and encourage them to cough while monitoring for any deterioration.

In severe airway obstruction, the player will have an ineffective cough. If they are unconscious, perform CPR. If conscious, alternate between back blows and abdominal thrusts.

Back blows are performed by standing behind the person and encouraging them to lean forward. Supporting their chest with one hand, sharply strike between the shoulder blades with the heel of your other hand. This should be repeated a maximum of five times before proceeding to abdominal thrusts. After each back blow, you must check to see if the obstruction has been expelled, in which case stop and reassess the airway.

Abdominal thrusts are carried out if back blows have been unsuccessful. Standing behind the person, place both arms around the upper abdomen. Make a fist with one hand and place between the player's

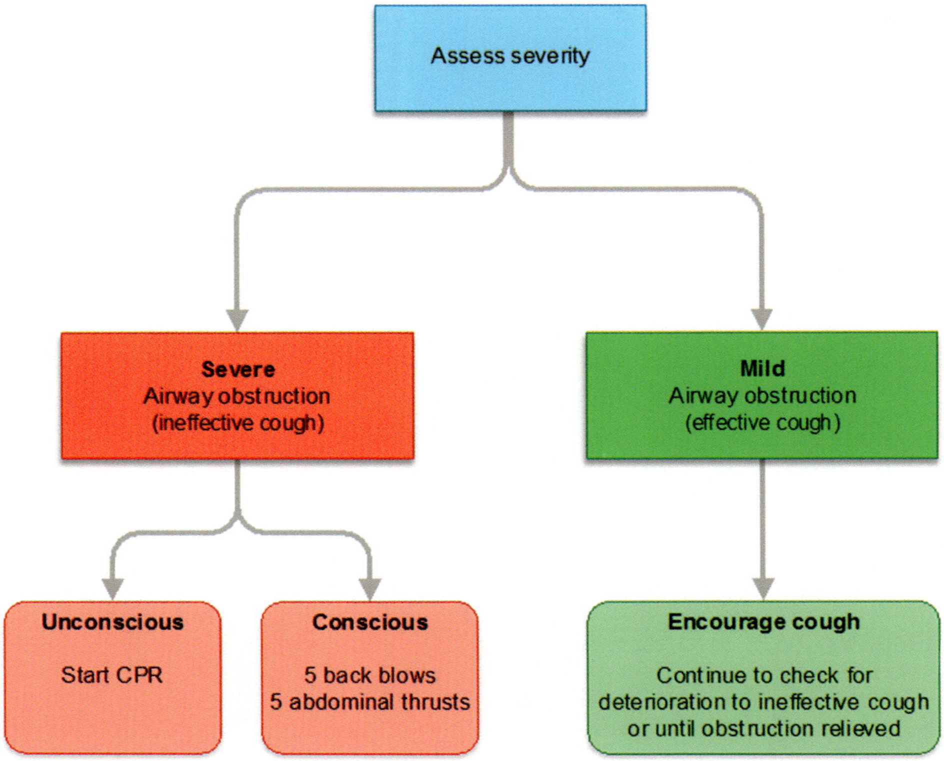

Fig. 2.9 Adult choking treatment algorithm. (Copyright European Resuscitation Council – www.erc.edu – 2016_NGL_043.)

umbilicus and xiphisternum. Grasp the clenched fist with your other hand and sharply pull inward and upward. Again, repeat a maximum of five times, checking each time to see if the foreign body has been expelled.

If the obstruction has not been relieved, then repeat the initial assessment and start again at back blows if required (**Fig. 2.9**).

Chapter 3

Medical Emergencies

Jonny Gordon

3

3.1 Anaphylaxis

Anaphylaxis is an immune response caused when a person is exposed to an allergen for the second time. This is a type I, immunoglobulin E (IgE) mediated response. An *anaphylactoid* reaction is clinically indistinguishable to this but does not occur as the result of an immune response.

Both conditions can produce life-threatening systemic changes that ultimately cause airway obstruction and circulatory collapse. Bronchial smooth muscle constricts causing bronchospasm, while vascular smooth muscle relaxes, and there is increased capillary permeability causing hypotension and potential shock.

3.1.1 Pathophysiology

In both anaphylaxis and anaphylactoid reactions, the antigen stimulates release of histamine, prostaglandin, and leukotriene from basophils and mast cells. The way in which this occurs varies between the two processes.

In **anaphylaxis**, the antigen initially stimulates production of IgE, which binds to the mast cells and basophils. When the antigen is reintroduced, it binds to the IgE already attached to the cells, resulting in an indirect release of chemical mediators from the cells.

In an **anaphylactoid** reaction, this release is usually the result of a direct binding of the antigen to the cells, or of activation of the complement system. IgE is not involved.

The end result of both processes is the same. Note that the term anaphylaxis will be used here to cover both types of reaction. Most reactions will occur within minutes of exposure to the allergen and usually within an hour. There may or may not be a previous history of anaphylaxis or allergy.

3.1.2 Common Allergens

Many allergens are commonly found, such as nuts, strawberries, and stings. From a prescribing viewpoint, it is imperative that you ascertain the allergy status of any players to whom you prescribe any medications. Nonsteroidal anti-inflammatory drugs (NSAIDs) such as ibuprofen or Voltarol and antibiotics such as the penicillin family are well known to have a side effect profile which includes allergy or anaphylaxis. In many of these cases, the player will be aware of the reaction they are having. It is the clinician's responsibility to ensure an appropriate history is taken prior to prescribing these medications.

Patients who suffer from asthma are recognized to experience more severe reactions and have a higher incidence of death from anaphylaxis, especially if there is a delay in administration of adrenaline. (Asthma should also be considered in the possible differential diagnosis of anaphylaxis.)

3.1.3 Clinical Manifestations

The clinical signs are all related to the effects of the mediators on the end organs (**Table 3.1**).

Assessment and management is according to your ABCDE assessment, i.e., treating any immediate or emerging life-threatening features in order. It is also important to remove the allergen if at all possible (remove the sting with forceps, for example).

3.1.4 Recognizing Anaphylaxis

The distinction between an allergy and anaphylaxis has been simplified such that anaphylaxis should be considered likely when all three of the criteria below are present:

- **Rapid progression of symptoms.**
- **Skin or mucosal changes in association with either.**
- **Airway compromise and/or respiratory compromise and/or circulatory compromise (i.e., decreased blood pressure [BP]).**

Skin changes vary from erythema to urticaria (similar in appearance to the rash of a nettle sting). Angioedema is a skin manifestation similar to

Table 3.1

Clinical manifestations of anaphylaxis

Body system	Clinical manifestation
Airway	Swelling of tongue or mucosal surfaces, e.g. lips; stridor, hoarseness
Breathing	Wheezing, increased respiratory rate; cyanosis is a late sign
Circulation	Tachycardia, hypotension, increased capillary refill time
Skin	Flushed, itchy, urticaria
GI	Diarrhea or vomiting

urticaria but involving deeper tissues such as submucosal or subcutaneous rather than the skin surfaces in urticaria.

Skin changes are present in the vast majority of cases of anaphylaxis but may be absent in up to 20% of cases.

In contrast, an allergy may occur with skin or mucosal changes, but without rapid progression or the associated A, B, or C system collapse.

Remember, in approximately 20% of patients suffering an anaphylactic reaction, there may be no skin changes. Also, skin changes in isolation are not diagnostic of anaphylaxis and so the entire clinical picture needs to be considered.

Diarrhea or vomiting may occur as part of the anaphylaxis reaction but neither is critical in terms of diagnosis. Many people believe themselves to be allergic to a medication when it is in fact a side effect rather than allergy.

See http://www.resus.org.uk/pages/reaction.pdf for more information on anaphylaxis.

3.1.5 Immediate Management of Anaphylaxis

This is summarized in the algorithm in **Fig. 3.1**. It is important to note that the system of assessment and treatment follows the ABCDE approach described earlier in Chapter 2. The immediate treatment will depend slightly on the experience of the clinician, the available equipment, and monitoring. It should be noted, however, that the algorithm clearly describes the initial treatment of the patient with adrenaline, chlorpheniramine, and hydrocortisone, all via the intramuscular (IM) route and therefore **no intravenous (IV) cannula is actually required for treatment to commence.**

Oxygen should not be forgotten, as it is the first drug given. It should be applied using a trauma mask with a reservoir bag and a maximum flow rate—usually 15 L per minute.

In anaphylaxis, lying the player down and elevating their legs is likely to be helpful only as a temporary measure. If this needs to be done, it indicates that the patient is likely to require IV fluids. The downside of someone lying down with their legs elevated is that if there are airway or breathing problems, they are far more likely to be trying to sit up to allow their body position to help with this.

Adrenaline

Adrenaline is given intramuscularly not intravenously. The dose administered IM is from 1:1,000 solution—0.5 mg in an adult = 0.5 mL IM 1:1,000. IV adrenaline only has a place in the treatment of an arrested player or a player under specialist care with full resuscitation equipment and monitoring. The dose is administered in the anterolateral aspect of the middle third of the thigh and can be re-administered after 5 minutes if there is no improvement in the player's condition.

Recent studies suggest it may be beneficial to use a blue or green needle in order to ensure the muscle is reached.

Autoinjectors may be carried by some athletes. It is vital that you are familiar with the past medical history of each player in order to know who is taking what medication, when, and why. Autoinjectors are no different, and being aware of any previous problems with anaphylaxis is a very useful first stage in being prepared to deal with them. A dose via autoinjector is either 0.3 or 0.15 mg.

Chlorpheniramine and Hydrocortisone

Use of these medications is theoretical rather than evidence based. They should be administered after the primary survey and treatments have already started as they will not affect the immediate course of the illness (first few hours). Steroids may be beneficial in shortening the course of the illness and this is especially true in patients with a past history of asthma.

3.1.6 Biphasic Reactions

These are difficult to predict and rebound may occur in anyone suffering from an anaphylactic reaction. Research would suggest hospital monitoring for at least 6 hours and possibly up to 24 hours in anyone who has previously suffered from a rebound reaction.

3.1.7 Referral

Although not specifically the remit of the sports physician, anyone in your care who has suffered from an anaphylactic reaction should be referred for specialist assessment to identify any specific triggering allergens. This may involve communication with the individual's general practitioner or directly with an immunologist.

EUROPEAN RESUSCITATION COUNCIL

Anaphylaxis

Anaphylactic reaction?

↓

Assess using ABCDE approach

↓

Diagnosis - look for:

- Acute onset of illness
- Life-threatening Airway and/or Breathing and/or Circulation problems[1]
- And usually skin changes

↓

- **Call for help**
- Lie patient flat with raised legs (if breathing allows)

↓

Adrenaline[2]

↓

When skills and equipment available:

- Establish airway
- High flow oxygen
- IV fluid challenge[3]
- Chlorphenamine[4]
- Hydrocortisone[5]

Monitor:

- Pulse oximetry
- ECG
- Blood pressure

---

[1] **Life-threatening problems:**
Airway: swelling, hoarseness, stridor
Breathing: rapid breathing, wheeze, fatigue, cyanosis, $SpO_2 < 92\%$, confusion
Circulation: pale, clammy, low blood pressure, faintness, drowsy/coma

[2] **Adrenaline** *(give IM unless experienced with IV adrenaline)*
IM doses of 1:1000 adrenaline (repeat after 5 min if no better)

Adult	500 mcg IM (0.5 mL)
Child more than 12 years	500 mcg IM (0.5 mL)
Child 6-12 years	300 mcg IM (0.3 mL)
Child less than 6 years	150 mcg IM (0.15 mL)

Adrenaline IV to be given **only by experienced specialists**
Titrate: Adults 50 mcg; Children 1 mcg kg^{-1}

[3] **IV fluid challenge (crystalloid):**

Adult	500 - 1000 mL
Child	20 mL kg^{-1}

Stop IV colloid if this might be the cause of anaphylaxis

	[4] **Chlorphenamine** (IM or slow IV)	[5] **Hydrocortisone** (IM or slow IV)
Adult or child more than 12 years	10 mg	200 mg
Child 6 - 12 years	5 mg	100 mg
Child 6 months to 6 years	2.5 mg	50 mg
Child less than 6 months	250 mcg kg^{-1}	25 mg

Fig. 3.1 Anaphylaxis algorithm. (Copyright European Resuscitation Council – www.erc.edu – 2016_NGL_043.)

3.2 Asthma

As with anaphylaxis, the incidence of asthma is documented to be on the rise in the general European population. Although it is a shared responsibility of the player and doctor to make sure the doctor is aware of any predisposing medical conditions the player may have, ASSUME this responsibility at the very start of your involvement with the team and make sure you are up to date with medical problems, ongoing injuries, and current medications.

Asthma is characterized by the triad of the following:

- Bronchoconstriction.
- Increased mucous production.
- Mucosal swelling due to inflammation.

Symptoms are classically coughing, wheezing, and breathlessness.

Precipitants are many and varied:

- Upper or lower respiratory tract infections.
- Exercise.
- Drugs—in sport, nonsteroidal anti-inflammatory medications such as ibuprofen or Voltarol are commonly prescribed and also well known to trigger bronchospasm.
- Poor compliance with treatment.
- Stress.
- Smoking.
- No specific trigger may be identified in many cases.

The main problem in treating the condition is in correctly identifying asthma as the diagnosis in the face of other differential diagnoses:

- Anaphylaxis.
- Pneumothorax.
- Pulmonary thromboembolism (PTE).
- Pulmonary edema—unlikely in sport but possible as part of altitude illness.
- Pneumonia.

The condition is likely to present in one of two ways:

- Very acute onset related to someone who has "brittle" airways disease with sudden onset of symptoms and little in the way of warning.
- More gradual deterioration in a player in whom asthma is known or suspected but who has not responded to treatment and who suddenly deteriorates.

3.2.1 Assessment of Acute Asthma

Use the ABCDE (Airway, Breathing, Circulation, Disability, Extraction from the field of play) approach in the initial assessment (see **Fig. 1.1**).

Depending on the severity of the attack, it may or may not be possible to take a history from the player. An **inability to complete sentences is a strong marker of severity and should be taken seriously.**

A: Are they breathing? (If not, then call for immediate help and follow cardiac arrest guidelines.) Consider checking for intraoral or mucosal swelling that may suggest an allergy or anaphylaxis as a differential.

B: Are there signs of any of the following?

- ✓ Cyanosis.
- ✓ Respiratory rate.
- ✓ Symmetry of chest movement.
- ✓ Accessory muscle use.
- ✓ Fatigue—anyone who appears fatigued or in whom the respiratory rate or respiratory effort is declining (without an overall associated improvement in their condition in all other ways) is likely to suffer an imminent respiratory arrest.
- ✓ Saturations—if available to you.

- Are they completing sentences?
- Is air entry bilateral?
- Are they wheezing (polyphonic expiratory sound)? **Absence of wheezing may suggest an inability to shift air in and out of the lungs. The silent chest may also suggest impending respiratory arrest.**

If slightly tachypnoeic but completing sentences, perform a peak expiratory flow rate test. This should be compared to the player's normal "best"—a figure you should be familiar with from assessing them at the start of your involvement with them.

C: Pulse rate

BP.

(Is the player cyanosed, hypoxic, or shocked?)

D: Are there any signs of hypoxia or obtundation?

Glasgow Coma Scale or Alert, Verbal, Pain, Unresponsive scoring system—anything less than 15 or Alert is of great concern.

Clinical examination allows you to categorize the presentation into either a moderate, acute/severe, or life-threatening exacerbation according to the British Thoracic/SIGN Guidelines of 2016 (**Table 3.2**).

3.2.2 Treatment of Acute Asthma

- Give **high-flow oxygen to all patients** with acute asthma where available.
- Commence **nebulized beta-2 agonist (e.g., salbutamol 5 mg)** preferably driven by oxygen rather than air. (An alternative to nebulizers is to multi-dose, with or without spacer devices. Multidosing

3

Table 3.2

Guide to levels of asthma severity

Moderate	Acute Severe	Life-threatening
	Any ONE of:	Any ONE of:
Increasing symptoms	PEF 33–50% best or predicted	PEF < 33% best or predicted
PEF 50–75% of best or predicted	Respiratory rate ≥ 25/min	SpO2 < 92%; Silent chest
No features of acute severe asthma	Heart rate ≥ 110/min	Cyanosis
	Inability to complete sentences in one breath	Poor respiratory effort; Arrhythmia
		Exhaustion
		Altered conscious level; Hypotension

Abbreviation: PEF, peak expiratory flow.

is used commonly in pediatrics instead of nebulizers and has a role in adults where nebulizers are not available.)

- In severe asthma or asthma where there has been a poor response to the initial nebulizer, **consider continuous nebulizers.**
- In severe or life-threatening asthma, consider adding **ipratropium bromide 0.5 mg** to the beta-2 agonist nebulizer.
- In **all cases of acute asthma, give oral prednisolone 50 mg daily for 5 days.**
- Routine prescription of antibiotics is unnecessary.

3.2.3 Asthma and World Anti-Doping Agency

All details provided in this section are taken from http://www.wada-ama.org. Please note that the WADA Prohibited list is regularly updated, and these definitions were taken from the January 2017 Prohibited List.

The mainstay of treatment for asthma is inhaled glucocorticosteroids with the use of beta-2 agonists for emergency or breakthrough symptoms only. It should be emphasized that the overuse of short- and long-acting bronchodilators (beta-2 agonists) has detrimental health effects.

Prohibited Status of β-2 Agonists and Glucocorticosteroids

Beta-2 Agonists

All beta-2 agonists (e.g., terbutaline, procaterol) not mentioned as exceptions below are prohibited and require a therapeutic use exemption (TUE).

Salbutamol. Inhaled salbutamol is no longer prohibited. However, the presence of salbutamol in the urine in excess of 1,000 ng/mL is presumed not to be a therapeutic use of the substance and will be considered as an adverse analytical finding. The athlete would then need to document the details of his/her medical condition and medication use. The athlete may then be required to prove, by a controlled pharmacokinetic study, that the abnormal test result was the consequence of the use of a therapeutic dose (maximum 1,600 mcg over 24 hours, not to exceed 800 mcg every 12 hours) of inhaled salbutamol.

Salmeterol. Inhaled salmeterol is no longer prohibited. The maximum inhaled dosage must not exceed 200 mcg over 24 hours.

Formoterol. Inhaled formoterol to a maximum delivered dose of 54 mcg over 24 hours is no longer prohibited. The presence in urine of formoterol in excess of 40 ng/mL is presumed not to be a therapeutic use of the substance and will be considered as an adverse analytical finding unless the athlete proves, through a controlled pharmacokinetic study, that the abnormal result was the consequence of the use of no greater than 54 mcg over 24 hours. If a dosage in excess of 54 mcg/d is legitimately required by the athlete, then a TUE must be requested.

Glucocorticosteroids

All glucococorticosteroids are prohibited when administered by oral, IV, IM, or rectal routes.

Prohibited treatments can only be provided to players when a TUE application has been **approved** in writing by the competent authority. TUE applications must be signed by the player and the prescribing doctor, and must be submitted to the correct authority (which will be **one** of FIFA, UEFA, or the relevant national antidoping organization, depending on the competition). Unless an emergency (i.e., life-threatening) situation, treatment should not be administered until the TUE is approved.

TUEs for asthma must be submitted with specific clinical evidence. Always consult the WADA website for the most up-to-date guidelines for the documentation required to support asthma submissions. The validity of a TUE for an asthmatic athlete is 4 years with at least annual confirmation of the treatment regime by a respiratory physician or a physician experienced in treating asthma in athletes. After 4 years, repeated pulmonary function tests must meet the agreed diagnostic criteria.

Other asthma medications NOT currently on the prohibited list are as follows:
- Leukotriene receptor antagonists.
- Anticholinergics.
- Sodium cromoglycate (chromones).
- Theophyllines (xanthines).
- Anti-IgE agents.

3.3 Seizures

The focus of management should be prevention in anyone with previous seizure activity.
Incidence of seizures in the general population is about 1%. The definition of epilepsy is variable. It is most commonly defined as a tendency to suffer from recurrent seizures.

3.3.1 Classification

By Cause

- Primary—idiopathic.
- Secondary—symptomatic.

By Clinical Features

Generalized Seizures. Epileptic activity involves both halves of the brain; consciousness is always lost.
- Grand mal:
  - Tonic-clonic.
  - Clonic.
  - Myoclonic.
- Petit mal:
  - Usually in children.
  - Otherwise known as "absence" seizures.

Partial Seizures. Epileptic activity involves part of the brain.
- Simple—no loss of consciousness.
- Complex—possible partial loss of consciousness or inability to remember aspects of the fit.

A partial seizure may progress to a generalized seizure and this is then known as a secondary generalized seizure.

Status Epilepticus. Seizure activity ongoing for more than 30 minutes or repeated seizures without consciousness being regained are life-threatening conditions with a high mortality, the rate of which increases with the increasing duration of the seizure.

3.3.2 Management Aims

- To maintain the airway.
- To terminate the seizure if not terminated within 2 minutes.
- To identify potential reversible causes of a secondary seizure—namely, **hypoglycemia**.

3.3.3 Secondary Causes of Seizure

At pitchside, it is vital to assess for potentially reversible causes of the seizure and to carry out simple measures. Important acute causes to be considered are the following:
- **Hypoglycemia**—easily the most important and the most likely to be reversed as long as it is identified (check blood glucose level in any fitting patient).
- **Trauma**—consider extradural hematoma or contusions after head injury.
- **Electrolytes**—hyponatremia or hypocalcemia.
- **Infection**—meningitis or encephalitis.

3.3.4 Medications

The administration of seizure-terminating medications of the benzodiazepine family will partly depend on the experience of the clinician and availability of the drug. Treatment can be delivered intravenously, as well as via other routes such as buccally or intranasally. Midazolam appears to be gaining favor, especially in the pediatric setting.
All members of the benzodiazepine family have similar side effects, such as respiratory depression and hypotension. The extent of these effects varies depending on the specific drug, but it is vital that you are familiar with these effects and are competent in the management of the airway (**Fig. 3.2**).
Compared with diazepam, lorazepam has an equivalent time of onset but a much shorter duration of action. The adult recommended dose is 4 mg (0.1 mg/kg in children). It can, however, be administered as 2 mg followed by a further 2 mg two minutes later if there is no initial response. After a further ten minutes, the same 4 mg dose can be repeated—either as a bolus of 4 mg or split into 2 mg plus a further 2 mg again after two minutes.

NOTE

Whatever you take in your medical bag, make sure you are familiar with the effects that administering it will have on your player.

If you are unable to check blood sugar in a fitting player, you should consider administering IV glucose as this is the only real reversible cause of a seizure that can be treated at pitchside. It is unlikely that the risks of this will outweigh the benefits. Indeed, it is possible that you will be unsuccessful in terminating a hypoglycemic seizure with benzodiazepine alone.

3.3.5 When to Phone an Ambulance?

- Status epilepticus.
- Player's first seizure.
- Seizure as a result of injury.

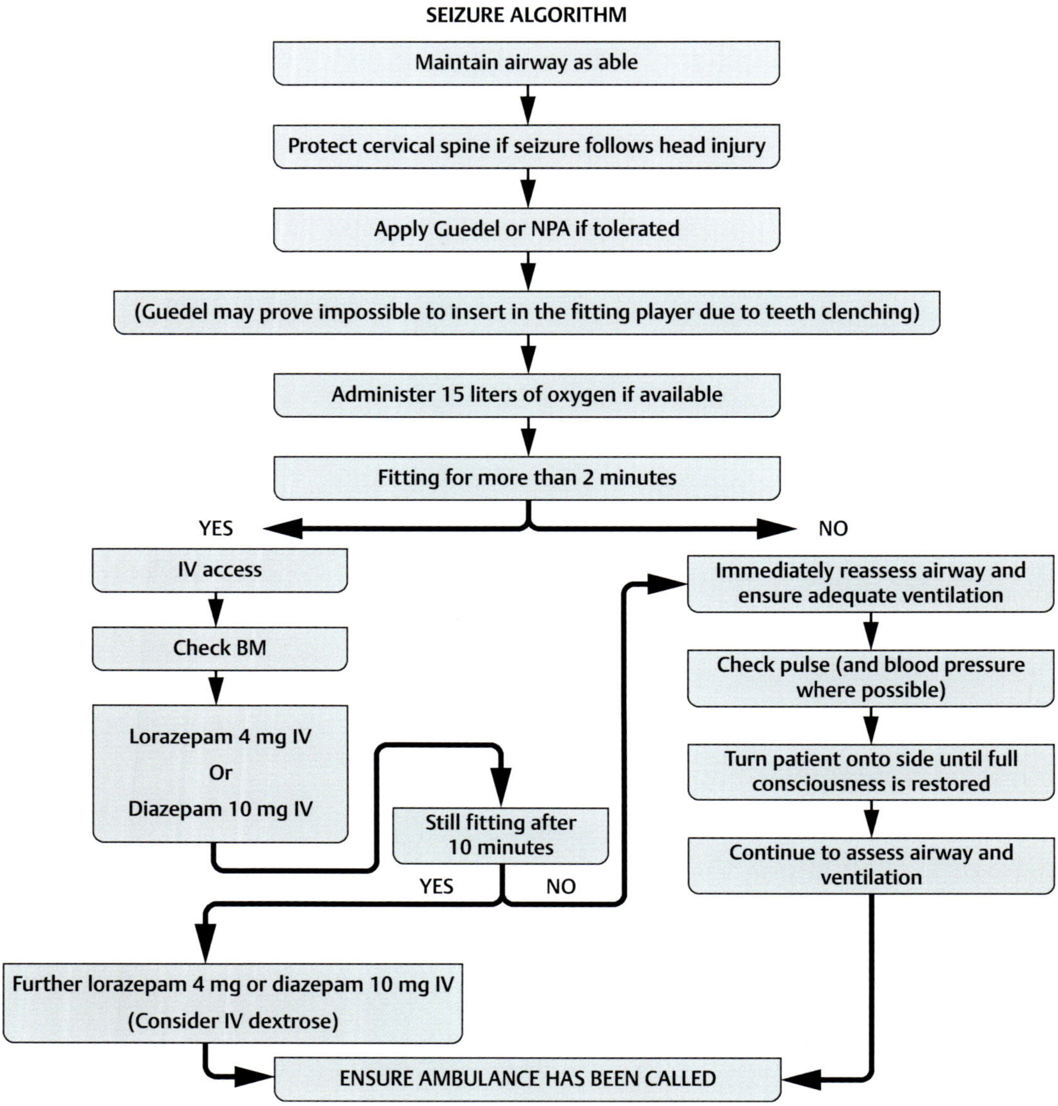

Fig. 3.2 Seizure algorithm.

- Injury resulting from seizure.
- Seizure lasts longer than 5 minutes.
- Multiple seizures.

3.4 Diabetic Emergencies

Diabetes is a condition that results from a lack of endogenous insulin resulting in fluctuating and elevated blood glucose levels.
Approximately 10 to 15% of all sufferers of diabetes worldwide are insulin-dependent, also known as Type 1, and 85 to 90% are noninsulin dependent (Type 2). The incidence is increasing in all age groups but most notably in Type 2 where dietary factors are attributed as a major cause. Exercise should actively be encouraged in patients who have diabetes.
Given the high prevalence of diabetes in our society, it is distinctly possible that you may be called upon to care for a player with the condition at some point during your time looking after a sports team.
As mentioned earlier, it is vital that you are aware of anyone in your care who has the disease, the medications that they take for this, and the problems and symptoms they usually suffer from.
You may be called upon to deal with a player suffering from the effects of diabetes who is either a known diabetic or presenting for the first time.

History of lethargy, polyuria, and polydipsia are the classically described symptoms for someone presenting with diabetes. In the context of tachycardia, hyperventilation and dehydration, diabetic ketoacidosis (DKA) should be considered. Similarly, any player suffering from a seizure or drop in their conscious level should also ALWAYS have their blood sugar tested.

The normal reference range is 4 to 6 mmol/L, though this can increase to 8 mmol/L after a meal. The blood glucose reading may be higher than this, however, and a fasting glucose or glucose tolerance test will usually be required to confirm the diagnosis.

3.4.1 Diabetes and World Anti-Doping Agency

Insulin is a prohibited substance on the World Anti-Doping Agency (WADA) Prohibited List and as such each player diagnosed with Type 1 diabetes must ensure they have a TUE certificate in accordance with WADA requirements.

The following substances and their releasing factors are prohibited (see www.wada-ama.org):

- Erythropoiesis-stimulating agents, e.g., erythropoietin (EPO), darbepoetin (dEPO), hypoxia-inducible factor (HIF) stabilizers, methoxy polyethylene glycol-epoetin beta (CERA), peginesatide (hematite).
- Chorionic gonadotrophin (CG) and luteinizing hormone (LH) in males.
- Insulins.
- Corticotrophins.
- Growth hormone (GH), insulin-like growth factor-1 (IGF-1), fibroblast growth factors (FGFs), hepatocyte growth factor (HGF), mechano growth factors (MGFs), platelet-derived growth factor (PDGF), vascular endothelial growth factor (VEGF), as well as any other growth factor affecting muscle, tendon or ligament protein synthesis/degradation, vascularization, energy utilization, regenerative capacity, or fiber type switching; and other substances with similar chemical structure or similar biological effect(s).

3.4.2 Hypoglycemia

A blood glucose level below 4 mmol/L is regarded as a hypoglycemic (hypo) event. This is an emergency because the brain is being deprived of energy. The causes of a hypo include the following:

- Too much insulin or sulphonylureas.
- Exercise.
- Not enough food.

Hypoglycemia may occur at any time, but there is a greater chance of this happening when exercising or before the next meal is due.

Symptoms

Features of a ***mild hypo*** include the following:

- Sweaty, pale, anxious, hungry, weak, trembling.
- Mood and behavior alteration (anxiousness or aggression).
- Poor coordination.

In a ***moderate hypo***, other signs develop, including the following:

- Headache, dizziness, difficulty concentrating, abdominal pain and nausea, visual disturbances.

In a ***severe hypo***, the signs progress to include the following:

- Inability to stand.
- Possible severe aggression/agitation.
- Loss of consciousness or seizures.

Treatment of Mild to Moderate Hypo

Treatment aims are to prevent progression from a mild episode to a severe one.

In mild to moderate hypo, the player is conscious and can be treated by giving sugary drinks or foods by mouth.

Important Points

- Do not leave anyone having a hypo alone. Someone needs to stay with the player at all times to ensure the hypo is successfully treated and there is no deterioration.
- A fast-acting carbohydrate should be given such as a sports drink, jelly sweets, or Hypostop.
- Repeat this treatment if there has been no response within 10 minutes.
- Follow up by giving slowly absorbed carbohydrate. This should be administered as soon as the player starts to recover having had the shorter acting sugars. Bananas, sandwiches, or biscuits will provide a more sustained release of carbohydrate.

Treatment of Severe Hypo

If the player is unconscious, perform an ABC assessment and have the player lie on their side if possible. Medical treatment for a severe hypo is either an IV injection of glucose or an IM injection of glucagon.

Glucose can be given in differing concentrations. The aim is to give 25 g either as 125 mL of 20% glucose or as 250 mL of 10% glucose. Glucose at 50% is irritant to the vein and should only be used if no alternative is available. The cannula should be flushed through immediately after.

There is no place to give a buccal glucose solution such as Hypostop to an unconscious or fitting athlete.

An alternative to IV glucose is IM glucagon 1 mg which takes about 10 minutes to act and can be given if IV access is going to be difficult to achieve.

If the player has symptoms and their reading is on the low side of normal, continue to treat as for a mild hypo. If you are approached by a player with a low reading but no symptoms, treat them—do not wait for symptoms to occur.

3.4.3 Hyperglycemic Crisis

DKA is a condition caused by lack of insulin—usually poor compliance.

The diagnosis of DKA should be made in a player with the following:

- Hyperglycemia (blood glucose > 14 mmol/L usually).
- A metabolic acidosis.
- Ketones in the urine, present on urine dipstick.

In the dressing room, you will be able to confirm the high blood glucose but you will not have access to biochemistry tests. A metabolic acidosis will be suggested clinically by the ongoing high respiratory rate of the player as they attempt to correct the build-up of the acid in the body. Ketones may be smelt on the athlete's breath suggesting ketonemia, but it is unlikely that you will be able to test their urine for ketones as they will likely be so dehydrated that they will be unable to pass urine without significant IV fluid replacement and probably a catheter.

Principles of management are to correct the dehydration, which is more life-threatening than the hyperglycemia. If you have access to IV fluids, then this is far more important than commencing insulin. Start a liter of crystalloid and transfer to hospital by ambulance. DO NOT give a bolus of insulin either IV or subcutaneously.

Chapter 4

Trauma Emergencies

Jonny Gordon

4

4.1 Spinal Injury

Initial assessment of any injured footballer always starts as a joint assessment of the airway **at the same time** as the cervical spine.

The cervical spine is affected in 55% of all spinal injuries. The remaining 45% is split equally between the thoracic, thoracolumbar, and lumbosacral spines.

The mechanism of injury is helpful in suggesting the type of pathology that will occur. For example, axial loading, which could be caused by falling from a height onto the head, is more likely to result in a burst fracture of the C1, whereas a hyperextension injury is more commonly associated with a fracture of the C2.

A fracture of the cervical spine is also associated with a 10% likelihood of spine fracture at another location.

The spine should be thought of in terms of the anatomy, physiology, and pathology. Maintaining normal anatomical alignment will help prevent the extension of any primary spinal injury. Ensuring that physiological problems such as hypoxia and hypotension do not occur will help prevent secondary complications such as spinal cord ischemia or edema —the causes of secondary cord injury.

4.1.1 Anatomy

The **spinal column** is the supporting structure that protects the cord. It consists of 7 cervical, 12 thoracic, 5 lumbar, and 5 sacral vertebrae, along with the coccyx. The vertebral bodies are located anteriorly and provide much of the strength of the column. The vertebral arch is posterior to the body and consists of two pedicles united posteriorly by the laminae. The function of the arch is to protect the spinal cord, which it encircles. The vertebral bodies are supported by strong ligaments anteriorly and posteriorly, while the intervertebral disks separate the vertebral bodies from each other.

The **spinal cord** runs from the medulla oblongata at the base of the skull down to about L1–L2 in the adult, terminating in the conus below which is the cauda equina. The cord can be injured at any point along its path, but the most devastating injuries occur in the cervical region as it is at this point that the nerves supplying the respiratory muscles are found. The spinal canal is relatively wide—most notably down to the level of the C2—and it is not until you reach the thoracic spine that the canal width decreases significantly. The increased risk to the cord at this area due to decreased physical space is offset purely by the limited mobility afforded by the thoracic spine due to the rigid thoracic cage. The areas where one part of the spine can act as a fulcrum against a more mobile adjacent area (namely, the cervicothoracic and thoracolumbar) are common sites of injury.

4.1.2 Classification of Injury

Injuries can be classified in a number of different ways:

- As primary or secondary.
- By the anatomical structures affected.
- By the level of cord injury.
- As complete or incomplete.
- By the association of hemodynamic collapse in the form of shock.

Remember, it is possible to have a spinal injury without a cord injury, so the absence of neurological symptoms or signs should not allow the neck to be cleared.

Primary versus Secondary Injury

A primary injury is an actual initial injury to the cord, usually caused by a direct compressive force from unstable bony architecture, i.e., fracture or subluxation. Our main goal is to prevent worsening of this by performing inline immobilization and securing the cervical spine.

Secondary injury is caused at cellular level by such factors as hypoxia or hypovolemia. Its effects can be minimized by administering high-flow oxygen and maintaining a systolic blood pressure (BP) of not less than 90 mmHg.

Anatomical Structures

At its most basic level, this can be divided into the affected anatomical region (cervical, thoracic, etc.). Specific fractures can occur at specific sites.

Cervical.

- *C1 (atlas)—Jefferson*: burst fracture, usually caused by axial loading.
- *C2 (axis)—odontoid peg fracture*: hangman's fracture, usually caused by a hyperextension injury.
- *C5:* the most common site of fracture.
- *C5/C6:* the most common site of subluxation.

Thoracic.

- *Wedge fracture:* occurs due to axial load with flexion; usually stable.
- *Burst fracture:* much more significant due to increased likelihood of bony fragment within the canal.

Lumbar.

- Again, may be wedge or burst fracture.
- Less likely to be significant than thoracic burst due to cord ending around L1.
- Injury around L1 may result in cauda equina syndrome.

Specific attention needs to be given to anyone with a cervical or high thoracic fracture, as their ventilatory status may decline if the muscles of respiration become paralyzed. The diaphragm is supplied by the phrenic nerve C3–C5, and dependency on the accessory and abdominal muscles may develop with "abdominal breathing," a highly concerning sign.

Level of Cord Injury

Note that the level of cord injury may differ from that of the bone injury, as the spinal nerves enter and exit the spinal canal and ascend or descend prior to entering the cord. The cord level is determined by clinical examination and is the lowest cord neurological level where the examination is normal on both sides of the body.

A number of different cord syndromes exist.

- **Central cord**—Usually the result of a forward fall onto the face. The central cord is supplied by the anterior spinal artery, and the pattern of neurology classically shows greater loss of power in the upper limbs compared with the lower. Recovery occurs with lower limbs resolving first. There can be variable sensory loss.
- **Cauda equina syndrome**—Nerve root pain in either or both legs with "saddle" anesthesia (i.e., around the anus), decreased anal tone, urinary retention, and bowel dysfunction.
- **Spinal cord injury without radiological abnormality (SCIWORA)**—Not a pitchside problem as this diagnosis is made once imaging has been completed by either computed tomography (CT) scan or X-ray. This highlights the ongoing level of concern that should be placed on the symptoms and signs and not just the imaging. SCIWORA is more prevalent in children due to their larger head-to-body ratio.

There are other cord syndromes, but it is not important that the nature of the type of injury is identified at pitchside—as long as focus is placed on correctly immobilizing the cervical spine.

Complete versus Incomplete Cord Injury

If motor or sensory function can be elicited at a region **below the level of the cord injury**, the patient has an incomplete injury.

Associated Neurogenic or Spinal Shock

In **neurogenic shock**, interruption of the sympathetic innervation of the heart results in bradycardia and hypotension. The heart cannot mount the usual tachycardia in response to hypovolemia and the BP will not respond to fluid. The player will be warm and hypotensive compared with an athlete suffering from hypovolemia, who will become progressively colder and hypotensive. Treatments include atropine and vasopressors.

Spinal shock is not shock as classically defined (failure to perfuse vital organs). It refers to the immediate loss of reflexes and flaccidity seen after cord injury with subsequent hyperreflexia found weeks after the injury.

The two terms "spinal shock" and "neurogenic shock" are not interchangeable.

4.1.3 Spine Assessment

Consider a cervical spine injury in anyone with the following:

- A head injury.
- An injury above the clavicles.
- A decreased Glasgow Coma Scale (GCS) score.
- A concerning mechanism of injury, e.g., fall while in midair, tackle where mechanism is unclear.

The cervical spine should be immobilized by gently holding either side of the head until the airway has been assessed. Assuming there is no issue with the airway, an assessment of the neck can then be made. Guidelines such as the Canadian Cervical Spine Rule published by Stiel et al in the Journal of the American Medical Association (JAMA) in 2001 suggest that the cervical spine can be considered "cleared" if the following criteria are met:

- **An absence of posterior midline cervical spine tenderness.**
- **A GCS of 15.**
- **An absence of focal neurological deficit—on motor or sensory testing.**
- **An absence of any distracting injuries.**
- **The ability to achieve *active* 45-degree lateral neck rotation in both directions.**
- **No concern over the mechanism of injury—such as an axial load to the head or a fall greater than 3 ft.**

A distracting injury is one deemed significant enough by the assessing clinician to cause so much pain as to distract the athlete from the possibility of recognizing that they also have a cervical spine injury—a long bone fracture, visceral injury, etc.

If all of the above criteria are met, then the neck can be "cleared" and hands removed from the head. If any of the above criteria are not met, then the cervical spine should be immobilized fully using an appropriately sized hard (also known as a semirigid) cervical collar and a scoop or a spinal board, with blocks applied to each side of the head and taped. The player should only be moved on and off the scoop or spinal board by logroll with sufficient people to assist. They should then be transferred to an appropriate hospital for imaging.

There can be confusion as to when the spine is considered fully immobilized. The cervical spine is considered immobilized in either of the following cases:

- The player has been placed on a scoop or a spinal board, a hard collar applied, the forehead taped onto the scoop or a spinal board (by placing tape across the board from one side of the board to the other across the forehead and over the chin), and sandbags or blocks have then been applied on either side of the head.
- Your hands are placed either side of the head to stop movement (with or without a hard collar on).

The neck is not considered fully immobilized if the player only has a hard collar on.

If you are unable to clear the spine for whatever reason, then you must remove the player for a more structured assessment away from the pitch, keeping the spine immobilized at all times.

4.1.4 Fitting a Hard or Semi-Rigid Collar

A number of these products are available and typically come in a variety of sizes. It is highly recommended that you use a single multiadjustable collar as this negates the need to carry round multiple collars of different sizes. The collar will typically come flat-packed and you should familiarize yourself with being able to construct the collar before you need to use it. Instructions are provided, but in terms of professionalism and reassuring the player, it is vital that you know how to size the collar before you need to use it on the pitch. Always fit according to the manufacturer's instructions.

The collar is usually sized by taking a measurement (in your fingerbreadths) from the angle of the player's mandible down to the "bulk of the trapezius muscle." This is the angle formed where the neck meets the trapezius (see **Fig. 4.1a**).

This equates to the same distance from the multiadjustable point on the collar down either to its lowermost plastic edge or to its sizing marker as is shown in **Fig. 4.1b**. This will depend on the type of collar and the manufacturer's instructions. If the collar is multiadjusting, then simply click it into position at the appropriate point (see **Fig. 4.1b**).

The collar is applied by sliding the flattest (posterior) part underneath the player's neck while someone else maintains control over the spine (**Fig. 4.1c**). The curved front of the collar can then be positioned across the front of the neck and secured with Velcro (**Fig. 4.1d**). The Velcro should never be forced into

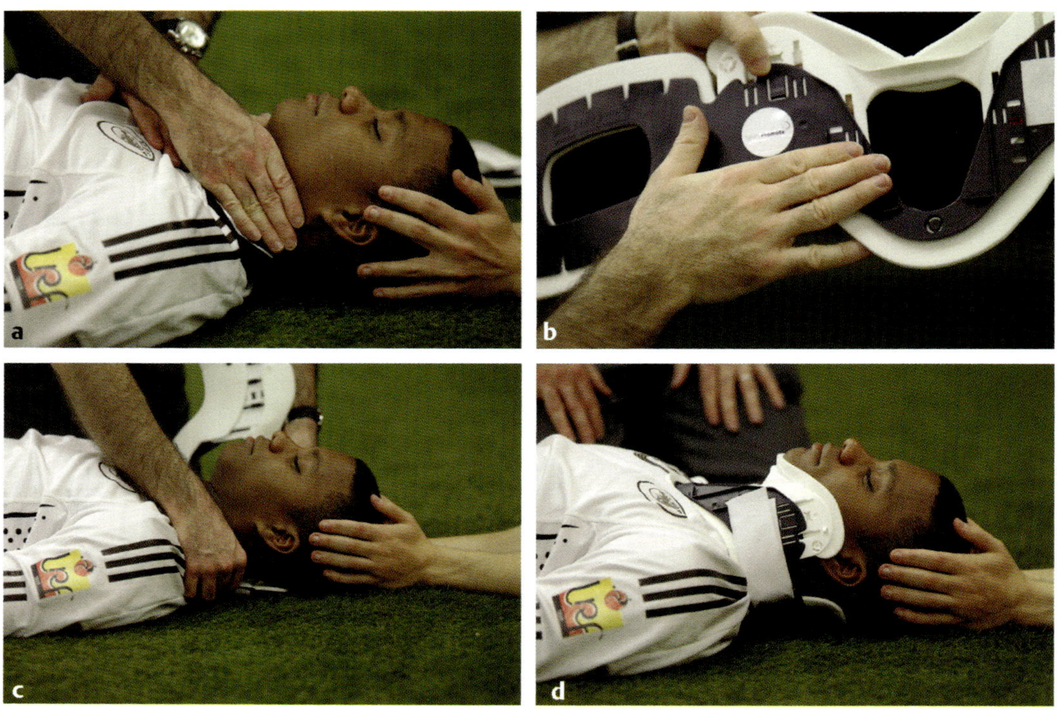

Fig. 4.1 Fitting a collar. **(a)** Measuring from the mandible to the bulk of the trapezius in fingerbreadths. (Note: the bulk of the trapezius is the point formed where the arrows meet.) **(b)** Sizing from the sizing point to the lowermost edge of (dark) plastic. (Note: the white is foam, not plastic.) **(c)** Sizing is made from the relevant multiadjustable point in the collar down to the sizing post (seen adjacent to the lowermost point of the ring finger). **(d)** Failure to apply a correctly sized collar can easily worsen the position of the neck and potentially cause movement of an unstable fracture.

position as this, in turn, could force the spine into an incorrect position.

4.1.5 Performing a Logroll

The increasing utilization of scoop stretchers and decline in the use of spinal boards has meant less emphasis has been placed on the skills required to perform a log roll. The log roll is however an important skill to acquire—it takes practice and an understanding of the impact on the spine if done incorrectly. A spinal board may be the only piece of extrication equipment you have and so knowledge of how to roll a patient onto it is important. The decision to perform a logroll should only be made once an ABC assessment has been carried out and the player has had an assessment of their cervical spine. Ideally a hard collar will have been applied, but this is not absolutely necessary as the team leader will have control of the spine during the roll.

The player should ideally already be positioned lying flat on the ground. If the hips are flexed, these should gently and gradually be lowered so that the legs and spine are in a straight line. The player's hands can be either placed across the chest or straightened out with the palms facing inward.

For an adult, the logroll requires four people to move the player and one to assess the spine and remove or place the spinal board.

Movers

The **leader** is at the head of the player and takes control of the head and neck (**Fig. 4.2a**). The three assistants stay on one side of the player who is rolled toward them (**Fig. 4.2b**). If there is an injury on one side (e.g., broken humerus), the assistants should be placed on the uninjured side.

In a situation where a player is to be turned from their back onto their right hand side, do the following:

- Chest—The first assistant reaches across the player's chest, placing one hand on the player's left shoulder and the other on the player's hip. Both hand are palm down (**Fig. 4.2c**).
- Pelvis—The second person places one hand on the player's waist just above the first assistant's hand (palm down). Their other hand is placed under the player's left knee (palm up; **Fig. 4.2d**).
- Legs—The third assistant places their left hand (palm up) under the player's left calf and their right hand under the ankle (**Fig. 4.2e**).

The leader will state at which point the player is to be turned over and to what extent—usually 90 degrees.

The leader should ensure everyone is versed in what will happen, and will initiate the roll by saying: "One, two, three, roll" (**Fig. 4.2f**). It is vital that everyone moves the player at the same time, so that the

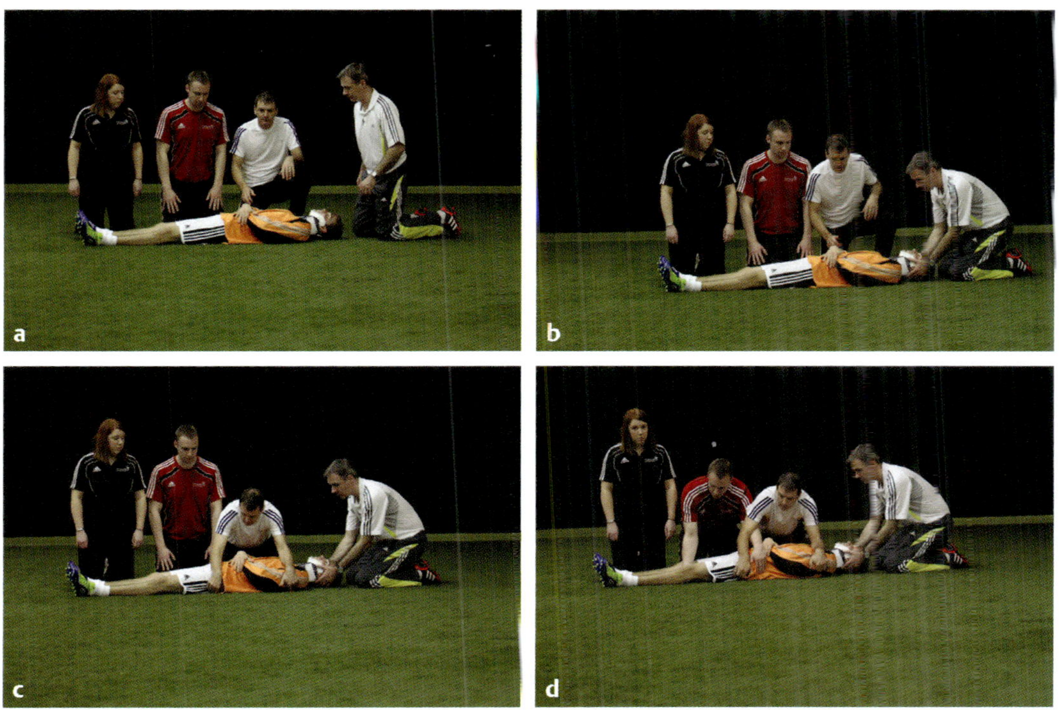

Fig. 4.2 Log roll. **(a)** Step 1. **(b)** Step 2. **(c)** Step 3. **(d)** Step 4.

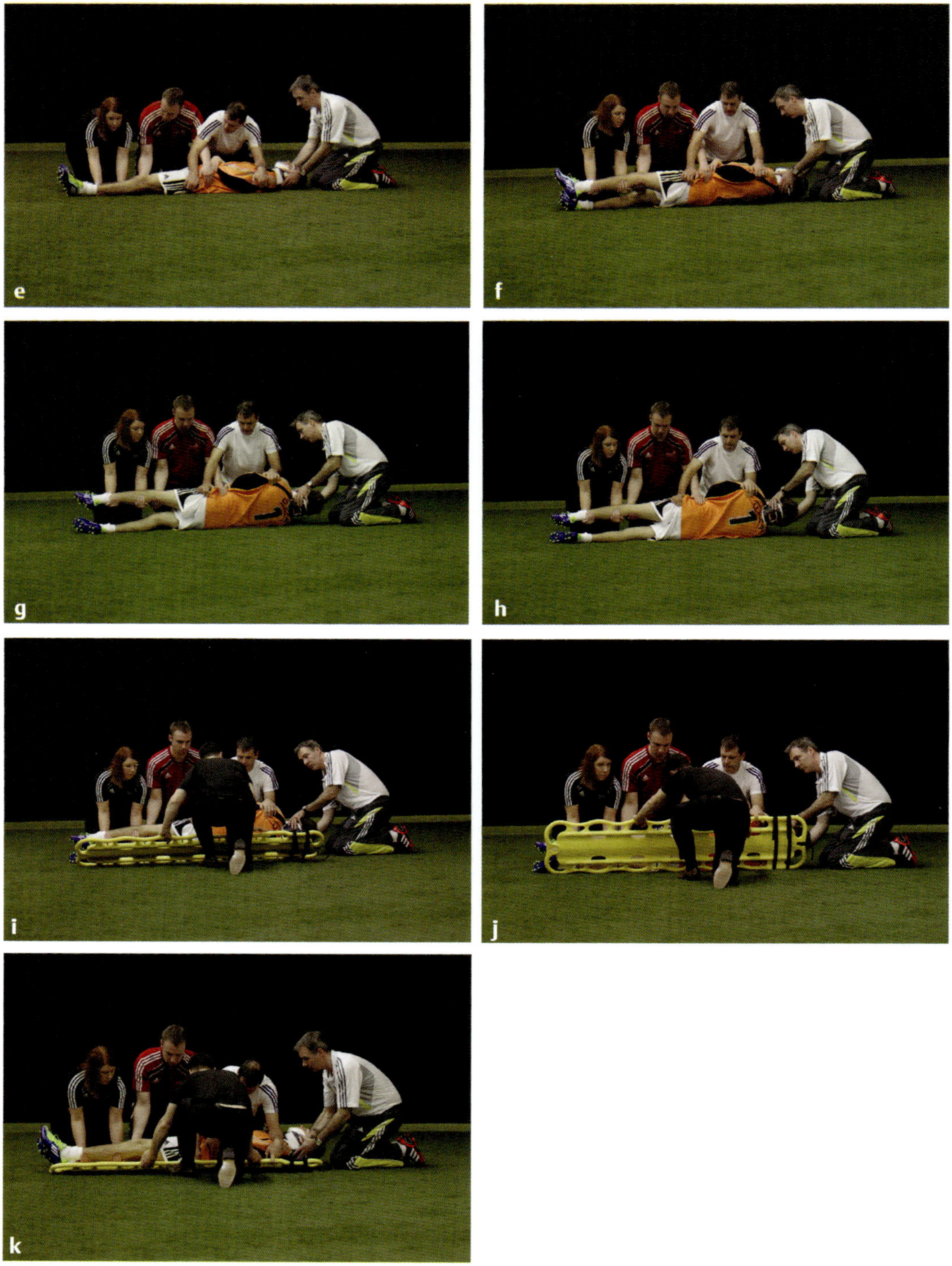

Fig. 4.2 *(continued)* **(e)** Step 5. **(f)** Step 6. **(g)** Step 7. **(h)** Step 8. **(i)** Step 9. **(j)** Step 10. **(k)** Step 11

spine effectively remains in a straight line at all times (**Fig. 4.2g**).

Once the player has been rolled to the optimum position, an assessment will be made by the fifth person (**Fig. 4.2h**). Once finished, the leader will again say: "One, two, three, roll," and the initial movement will be reversed so that the player is lying flat on their back again—with or without the spinal board having been moved into position by the fifth person (**Fig. 4.2i**).

Note that it is not necessary to move the patient through 90 degrees just to get the spinal board underneath them. The assistants have to watch the leader and take their cues about how far the player should be rolled (**Fig. 4.2j** and **Fig. 4.2k**).

Assessor

The assessor will be able to examine the spine once the player has been rolled onto his side. A quick but thorough look and palpation of the thoracolumbosacral spine is necessary. This will give an idea of the site of any tenderness, swelling, bruising, or palpable deformities. If an athlete has a head injury, remember to have a look at the occiput at the same time, as any wounds will be hidden once lying flat. Once finished, the assessor can either move a spinal board into position or remove the board as in the hospital setting.

Modified Logroll

It is acceptable to perform a logroll with only three movers and one assessor, when instead of three assistants there are only two. This can be done safely with a smaller person or child and may be necessary if there are only a few trained people available to help.

In the situation described earlier (logroll to the player's right-hand side), the first assistant would place their left hand onto the player's shoulder and their right hand on the player's left hip. The second assistant would place their left hand on the player's wrist and their right hand on the lower leg. This is not as satisfactory as a three-assistant maneuver, but is still acceptable in the cases described above.

What to Do If the Player Is Already Face Down

This is a difficult situation because of the possibility of associated airway compromise. Here, the leader positions their hands on the player's head such that they are already crossed over, i.e., imagine taking a beach ball and turning it upside down. This way, as long as the athlete is turned in the correct direction, the leader's hands will also uncross as the player moves through 180 degrees. In this situation, the other option is to use a second leader who can take control of the head when the roll reaches 90 degrees.

NOTE

In the setting of the pitchside assessment, all that actually matters is identifying the potential for injury, protecting the spine, maximizing the hemodynamic status (by doing simple things such as applying high-flow oxygen), and early definitive transfer.

4.2 Head and Facial Trauma

Head injuries are prevalent in certain sports and caution must be exercised when assessing these injuries especially if the player is to be returned to play. As detailed above, the structured assessment is key to ensuring injuries are not missed. Any head injury requiring treatment will by definition require the airway and cervical spine to be assessed as well. If there is any doubt at all about the conscious level, cervical spine immobilization procedures should be followed and the player should be removed from the field of play.

The Consensus Statement on Concussion in Sport from the Fourth International Conference on Concussion in Sport held in Zurich in November 2012 has been adopted by FIFA and contains information regarding return-to-play guidelines and assessment of concussion.

4.2.1 Anatomy

The bones of the skull are divided into those of the cranium and those of the face (**Fig. 4.3**).

- The cranium is further subdivided into the vault and the skull base.
- The vault is the aspect of the skull that overlies the brain. It comprises the frontal, parietal, squamous temporal, and occipital bones.
- The base of the skull is the lowermost portion of the skull—the area of the skull upon which the brain rests. It consists of the sphenoid and ethmoid bones, the mastoid and petrous portions of the temporal bone, and finally the base of the occipital bone.
- The face consists of the midface and jaw.
- The midface consists of the zygomatic, maxilla, nasal, lacrimal, vomer and palatine bones.
- The jaw is comprised solely of the mandible.

4.2.2 Types of Head/Brain Injury

Extracranial

Scalp Wounds

This is the most common wound you are likely to be required to treat in football.

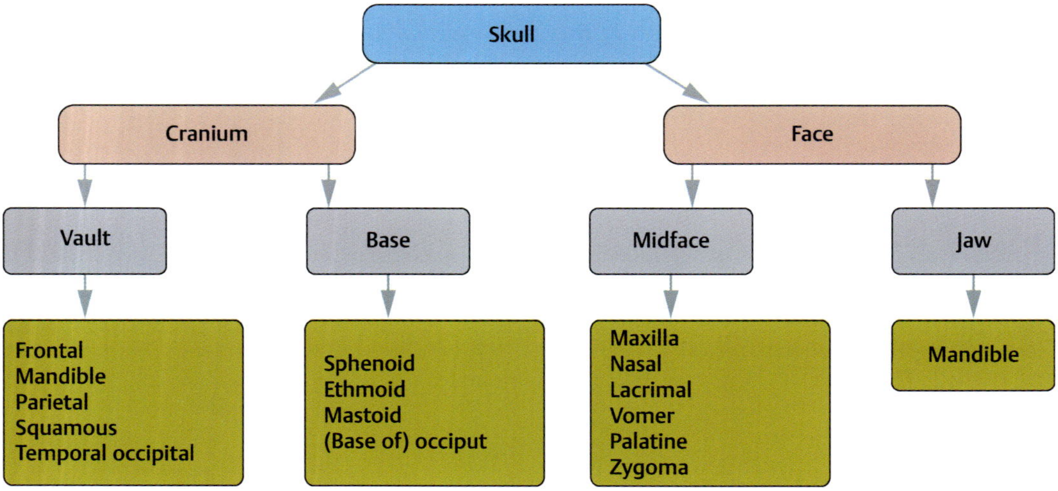

Fig. 4.3 Bones of the skull.

The anatomy of the scalp should be thought of in terms of the following:

- **S: skin.**
- **C: connective tissue.**
- **A: aponeurosis.**
- **L: loose connective tissue.**
- **P: periosteum.**

The scalp is highly vascular, which is beneficial in terms of healing and infection but also has the potential for significant bleeding. The aponeurosis or galea is a thin tendon-like tough sheet of tissue that attaches laterally to the temporal fascia and connects the frontal and occipital aspects of the occipitofrontalis muscle. There is potential for a space to form beneath this, and if the galea is not closed over when suturing a full-thickness scalp wound, a significant extra cranial collection may occur, which can become infected and require operative removal. The galea itself is so tough that when you assess a full-thickness scalp wound it may appear that you can feel a depressed skull fracture, when in fact you are feeling the torn galea.

There are many ways to treat a scalp wound during a competitive game, and these will be discussed as part of the course itself. **You must make sure that you are completely happy with your assessment of the entire player and not just the wound. Ultimately, it is not a bleeding scalp wound that is going to cause problems, but failure to assess and manage risks associated with the intracranial (IC) aspects of their head injury because of time spent patching up the laceration.**

If a player has a bleeding scalp wound, this should be assessed and treated as part of the circulation assessment, i.e., perform your A and B assessment first. Direct pressure applied to the wound is a vital first step. In fact, as long as you are carrying a gauze swab with you onto the pitch, you are likely to be in a position to manage most problems.

If you have never been taught to perform a procedure (e.g., suture), do not start at pitchside—remove the player to a place of safety and call for help.

Skull Fracture

Skull fractures are common sequelae to head trauma and therefore a common cause of morbidity. In isolation, they are not usually a direct cause of mortality unless they cause a catastrophic depression of the vault directly into the brain. This is exceptionally rare and would only occur as the result of a very high-impact collision—more the realms of a high-speed road traffic accident than a "traditional" footballing injury.

Direct mortality from head injury is usually the consequence of bleeding that occurs **with or without a skull fracture.** It is this associated bleeding that causes an increase in the IC pressure and ultimately brain herniation if this pressure is not released.

Linear Skull Fracture. This is common, especially in children. A linear skull fracture is a relatively straight-line break in the skull. In itself, it is not a serious injury unless there is an additional injury to the brain itself.

Depressed Skull Fracture. This type of fracture usually results from blunt trauma (e.g., from a knee) causing a dent to the skull. Such injuries can result in depressions of the bone into the brain. Depending on the depth of the depression, surgical intervention may be required to elevate the fracture fragment.

Basal Skull Fracture. This is a fracture usually resulting from significant force applied to the bones of the base of the skull. A classic physical appearance may appear with periorbital bruising (raccoon eyes) or

Battle's sign characterized by tracking bruising over the mastoid (i.e., bruising not as a consequence of direct trauma to the mastoid area). Leakage of fluid from the cerebrospinal fluid (CSF) spaces may result in rhinorrhea or otorrhea. Although a possible source of infection tracking back into the CSF, meningitis is actually very rare after a base of skull fracture and antibiotics are not currently recommended for prophylaxis of infection.

Intracranial

Extradural Hematoma

The dura is a thick, fibrous membrane that covers the brain and extends inferiorly through the foramen magnum. It is the outermost of the three meninges (dura, arachnoid, and pia mater) and divides into two layers. The middle meningeal artery lies between the two layers of the dura, and it is usually bleeding from this vessel that results in an extradural collection of blood. The bleeding fills a space between the dura and the internal table of the skull. The skull cannot expand and, as a result, the bleeding causes the dura to compress inward against the brain. Because of its relative thinness as a bone, and the position of the middle meningeal artery beneath it, trauma to the temporal area is the most likely cause of an extradural hematoma.

The "classic" clinical picture is one of the players having a lucid period prior to the pressure building to a critical point, at which time they will collapse. Timely neurosurgical intervention is required in all but the smallest of cases.

Subdural Hematoma

A subdural hematoma arises from bleeding between the potential space of the dura and the brain as opposed to the extradural which is bleeding between the skull and the dura. The origin of the bleed is usually bridging veins sheared and torn in this potential space. A footballer suffering from this injury will have an acute subdural which will develop suddenly. This is in comparison with the chronic subdural often seen classically in elderly patients who have had relatively minor trauma but become gradually confused as a result of the slowly expanding bleed. Again, neurosurgical intervention is likely to be required. The job of the team clinician is to ensure that maximum efforts are directed toward ensuring that secondary brain injury is minimized.

Subarachnoid Hemorrhage

Bleeding between the arachnoid and the closely adherent pia mater overlying the brain results in a subarachnoid hemorrhage. This may occur as a result of trauma, although it would be rare to find this in isolation without another type of bleed (either extra or subdural or even contusions). This type of presentation may also occur without trauma, as the result of a rupture of a "berry" aneurysm of the arteries supplying the brain. The player may collapse without warning or complain of a sudden headache, "as if someone has just hit me on the back of the head with a baseball bat." In view of this presentation of headache, a CT scan and a lumbar puncture would be required and therefore hospital transfer is necessary.

Other symptoms the player may complain of are neck stiffness, vomiting, or photophobia, which may make the diagnosis difficult to distinguish from meningitis. Management involves minimizing secondary brain injury, analgesia, and transfer to hospital.

Cerebral Contusion

A contusion is bleeding into the brain tissue itself and can be likened to a brain bruise. With the advent of modern CT and magnetic resonance imaging the diagnosis of these lesions has become much more commonplace, whereas in the past the symptoms were probably attributed to concussion. The management of cerebral contusions is usually nonsurgical unless there are other IC problems that require operative fixation (**Table 4.1**).

4.2.3 Pitchside Assessment of Players with Head Injuries

Ascertaining a history is vital when assessing a player with a head injury. If a player is unconscious when you arrive by their side, management can be relatively straightforward.

Perform an ABC assessment and protect their cervical spine.

They should not be returned to the field of play and will require assessment in hospital.

The framework for initial assessment should be followed and the player should be managed with oxygen, airway techniques if appropriate, cervical spine immobilization, and removal from the pitch on an

Table 4.1

Association of Glasgow Coma Scale (GCS), skull fracture, posttraumatic amnesia (PTA) and intracranial bleeding

GCS	Associated features	Risk of operable intracranial bleeding
15	No other features	1:31,000
15	With PTA	1:6,700
15	Skull fracture	1:81
9–14	No skull fracture	1:180
9–14	Skull fracture	1:5
3–8	No skull fracture	1:27
3–8	Skull fracture	1:4

appropriate extrication device such as a scoop or a spinal board.

If the player is fully conscious when you get to them, then again assess the cervical spine and take a history to elicit whether or not there has been a brief episode of loss of consciousness. An assessment should be made to ensure they are "topline" in the Alert, Verbal, Pain, Unresponsive (AVPU) or Glasgow Coma Scale (GCS) scoring systems. It does not matter which scoring system you use as long as you are thoroughly familiar with it. Anything less than "Alert" or GCS 15 mandates removal from the pitch and a hospital assessment.

If the ABCs are fine, the player is "Alert" or GCS 15 and there are no neurological symptoms or signs, an assessment should be made as to whether or not the player is fit to return to the field of play.

A series of questions should be asked of the player to ensure their "topline" mental status, and that no subtle confusion is present. The **modified Maddocks questions** are typically used in this situation:

- What venue are we at?
- What half is it?
- Who scored last?
- When did you last play?
- Did we win the last game?

These questions form a part of the Sport Concussion Assessment Tool 3 (SCAT 3) assessment published as part of the Zurich Consensus Guidelines.[1] The main difference in sideline assessment between SCAT 2 and the updated SCAT 3 (**Appendix I**)[2] is that the update puts more emphasis on simply recognizing potential symptoms and signs of concussion. The aim is clearly to ensure that the player is given the best opportunity to convey any subtle symptoms of concussion he may have—symptoms that may previously have been dismissed as trivial. For medicolegal purposes as well as consistency of assessment, it is highly recommended that you use the SCAT 3 sideline assessment to assess for concussion (see **Appendix II**).[1]

A failure to answer any of the modified Maddocks questions correctly suggests possible concussion and prevents a return to sport until a further detailed assessment has been made. If the player answers all the questions correctly and has not had a period of loss of consciousness, an assessment of balance and coordination can be made.

Take your time helping the player to stand, as standing too quickly is likely to result in dizziness and may make it difficult for you to know whether this is a result of the head injury.

While walking off the pitch with the player, a final decision will need to be made as to whether they are fit to come back on.

At the touchline, ask them again if they feel OK. Ensure they feel their vision is normal and check eye movements, assessing for double vision. Make sure both pupils react normally. **Note**: The tandem balance test as described in SCAT 2 has now been removed as part of the pitchside assessment due to the concern that muscle fatigue from exercise may give false positive results. It is advised that this is not performed now until at least after 15 minutes after the injury and is then compared against a baseline score.

You now have a player who has sustained a head injury, but:

- Has not lost consciousness.
- Has not suffered a seizure.
- Has been "Alert" or GCS 15 **at all times**.
- Has had a normal gross neurological assessment.
- Has answered modified Maddocks questions normally.
- Has normal balance.
- Has normal vision.
- Is asymptomatic.

You must keep a close eye on this player's movement, coordination, and the emergence of any other concerning features. If there is any doubt in your mind, then let the manager know and ask for the player to be substituted.

If a player has been removed from the field of play as the result of a head injury, **it is vital** that they are not left alone so that if they suffer a collapse or seizure or have a change in their symptoms, this can be managed immediately.

Indications for referral to hospital[3] are as follows:

- GCS of lower than 15 at initial assessment.
- Posttraumatic seizure.
- Focal neurological signs.
- Loss of consciousness.
- Severe and persistent headache.
- Repeated vomiting (two or more episodes).
- Posttraumatic amnesia of longer than 5 minutes.
- Retrograde amnesia of longer than 30 minutes.
- High-risk mechanism of injury (significant fall).
- Signs of skull fracture—CSF from nose or ears, hemotympanum, boggy hematoma, postauricular bruising, periorbital bruising).
- Coagulopathy.

4.2.4 Facial Trauma

Injuries to the face can cause significant problems in terms of the associated airway compromise, primarily in terms of a fracture of the midface or larynx, for example. Any injury to the face may also result in concussion, with or without an associated head injury, giving rise to a secondary airway obstruction from loss of protective reflexes due to obtundation.

It should be remembered that concussion can be caused by a transmissive force from any part of the body but, given the close proximity of the face to the head, it is not uncommon to suffer concussive symptoms purely as a result of a facial injury.

In any facial injury, an assessment for associated cervical spine injury should be made.

Principles of Managing Maxillofacial Injuries

History

Ascertaining the mechanism of injury is important. Think about associated complications such as neck pain or concussive symptoms. Is there any visual deficit—diplopia or visual loss? Is there numbness of the face suggesting an infraorbital nerve injury?

Examination

Start with an ABC assessment, clearing the cervical spine initially if possible. The face is a highly vascular structure, so make sure you have gloves and gauze swabs to allow you to apply direct pressure to any lacerations or nosebleeds. The primary aim of examination is to identify fractures and any associated cranial nerve injuries especially injuries potentially involving the facial or trigeminal nerves (**Table 4.2**).

Observe any wounds or hematomas. Is there any facial asymmetry from either localized swelling or bony depression caused by a malar complex fracture? Look in the mouth for bruising, broken teeth, or malocclusion. Any broken teeth must be accounted for and as such, a chest examination and even chest X-ray may be required if there is any suggestion of aspiration.

Palpate for evidence of a facial or even skull fracture. Systematically assess both sides of the face at the same time for comparison. Feel for a step at the infraorbital margin. Palpate the mandibular condyles. Assess for paresthesia below the eyes suggesting infraorbital nerve injury.

Table 4.2

Motor function testing for facial nerve damage

Facial nerve branch	Test of motor function
Frontalis	Look up/frown
Zygomaticotemporal	Close eyes tightly
Buccal	Wrinkle nose
Mandibular and cervical	Purse the lips

Assess eye movements and ensure no diplopia especially on upward gaze. Assess jaw movements and bite.

4.2.5 Soft-Tissue Injuries

Lacerations

All wounds need to be thoroughly examined to ensure that debris is removed and no contaminants remain. This is almost impossible to do at pitchside. There is very rarely an indication to patch up a bleeding wound at pitchside and return the player to the match without closing the wound properly. Remember that an assessment for concussion should also be carried out prior to returning the player to action. It is easy to focus on managing only one aspect of the injury and forgetting about another.

All facial wounds need to be closed with the aim of minimizing both the risk of infection and the extent of scarring. Any wounds must be thoroughly cleaned and explored prior to closure—usually with fine Ethilon or equivalent monofilament sutures. Glue may be an option with or without Steri-Strips. There is no place for the use of staples on the face.

Special Areas

Eye

The eyebrow is a common site of injury due to the prominent supraorbital ridge being injured during a clash of heads. Never shave off the eyebrow, as regrowth varies. Instead, use the eyebrow to align the edges of the wound to minimize the effect of any scarring. Eyelid wounds are rare in football and may need specialist involvement to close.

Mouth

Lacerations involving the vermilion border must be carefully apposed to minimize the cosmetic effect of any scar. A discrepancy of 1 mm or more will be noticeable at a conversational distance, so if you are unhappy about how a wound looks, start again. Wounds that are full thickness and extend through from the inside to the outer lip are usually closed externally and left to heal by secondary intention on the internal surface. Good oral hygiene is required. The tongue rarely ever needs to be sutured and this should not be performed at pitchside. Again, good oral hygiene is advised.

Hematomas

These are common injuries in football and are managed conservatively as long as an underlying bony injury is excluded either clinically or radiologically.

Pulsatile hematomas overlying structures such as the temporal artery should raise the suspicion of an underlying aneurysm, and lead to a referral for investigation. These may not appear immediately after an injury or may present as hematomas that fail to resolve fully.

4.2.6 Facial Fractures

Nasal Fracture

This is a very common injury and almost always the result of a clash of heads or collision between face and elbow.

Initial management is to stem any concurrent bleeding—with direct pressure where possible. It is important to assess for clinical deformity and signs of a septal hematoma, which is a maxillofacial emergency and needs urgent drainage to ensure the septum does not erode through. Associated wounds overlying the nasal bridge need to be thoroughly cleaned though antibiotics are not required, even though the fracture is technically compound.

Specialist review is required once swelling settles usually within 5 to 7 days.

Zygomaticomaxillary Complex Fractures—Malar Complex Fractures

Fractures of the zygomaticomaxillary complex (ZMC) are the second most commonly occurring facial fractures behind nasal fractures. The central portion of the ZMC is the malar prominence, and from this central area there are four attachments to the skull: the first connects to the frontal bone superiorly, the second connects laterally via the zygomatic arch to temporal bone, medially there is a connection to the maxillary bone and, lastly, there is a deep attachment to the greater sphenoid bone. The infraorbital margin can be fractured in isolation, as mentioned below, resulting in clinical signs of a blowout. It may also be fractured as part of a tripod fracture. In the situation of a tripod fracture (and where the zygomatic arch is broken in isolation), there may be a flattening of the facial features rather than marked swelling. The player will certainly require imaging and may require surgical elevation of the depressed fracture. As with those suffering a fractured orbit, advise the player to refrain from nose-blowing.

Orbital Fractures

These may occur as a consequence of direct contact with an opponent (e.g., elbow).

The important aspects of examining an injury to the eye relate to the resulting lack of function of the eye itself. You **must assess visual acuity** in anyone presenting with an eye injury and record the result of this assessment in their notes. Ensure the player can look upward without resulting double vision in the affected eye. Failure of this test is the result of the inferior rectus muscle entrapment caused by an orbital fracture. In a child, this will result in irreversible ischemia unless urgently operated on, making it a maxillofacial emergency. In an adult, this ischemia does not occur and there is no such urgency for the maxillofacial review. Similarly, assess for decreased sensation over the cheek or numbness of the upper gums, as this suggests involvement of the infraorbital nerve and again would necessitate expert review —usually within a week or so. Advise the player to refrain from blowing their nose.

The pupils should be assessed to ensure they are both reacting normally. Traumatic mydriasis occurs due to direct trauma to the eye, causing a rupture to the sphincter pupillae muscle. The pupil is dilated in comparison with the other eye, although it will still constrict slightly when light is shone into it. It is vital to assess for a hyphema in these situations (as in anyone with a direct eye injury). This is bleeding into the anterior chamber of the eye. In isolation, this may resolve within a week or so, but urgent ophthalmological assessment is vital to ensure pressures within the eye do not rise.

Mandibular Fractures

Mandibular fractures require a significant force and initial management should be based on assessing ABCs and the cervical spine. Fractures tend to occur in more than one place due to the ring-like structure of the mandible. Depending on the site of the fractures, the player may present with symptoms of pain, malocclusion, or paresthesia of the lower lip and chin. There may be an obvious deformity but signs can also be lacking and there may only be pain on opening the mouth in the case of undisplaced fractures. Look for intraoral bruising and assess the external auditory canal for evidence of bleeding, which would suggest the condyle has been forced upward into the canal. Assess for tenderness over the condyles and palpate the ramus, angle, and body of the bone. Analgesia will be required and the player should be referred to a maxillofacial specialist for operative repair in almost all cases. Where there is an injury affecting the tooth and the mandible, this should be considered a compound injury, and given the bacteria residing in the oral cavity, antibiotics are indicated.

Mandibular Dislocation

This can occur as the result of trauma or from rather more innocuous mechanisms such as yawning. It may be unilateral or affect both condyles. The player will be unable to close their mouth or swallow saliva properly. Relocation may be attempted (especially after Entonox analgesia) by standing in front of the player, placing your fingers in their mouth using swabs to protect them, and applying slow downward pressure to the molars in an inferoposterior direction.

4.2.7 Dental Injuries

Dental injuries occur commonly in football and may be associated with bony injuries such as mandibular fractures with malocclusion. Teeth may be completely avulsed, subluxed, or fractured.

The major issue arising from fractured or lost teeth is the risk of aspiration, and careful questioning and respiratory examination may be required to ensure this is not overlooked. The player should be asked to run their tongue over their teeth as this is one of the most sensitive ways to identify a new injury.

Avulsed teeth are a dental emergency as replacement should take place within an hour to ensure maximum chance of reimplantation. The tooth should only be held by the crown to minimize damage to the periodontal ligament. Do not clean unless there is heavy contamination with debris, in which case gentle cleaning with a saline solution or water may be useful.

The available options are the following:

- To replace into the socket and ask the player to bite down on gauze swabs for about 30 minutes—ideally en route to a dentist.
- To place the tooth in the mouth between the gum and cheek and transfer to a dentist. This should obviously only be done in situations when the player is fully conscious.
- To place the tooth in a container of milk and transport to a dentist.

Fractured teeth can be painful but do not require further pitchside treatment other than analgesia and referral for dental review.

Subluxed teeth should be placed back in as normal a position as possible. Again, a dental review should be arranged.

Dental injuries could be more easily prevented with the use of mouth guards. Even in situations where mouth guards do not protect from a fracture, they act as an area where the teeth remain, allowing an increased chance of reimplantation while minimizing the risk of aspiration.

4.3 Chest Trauma

Injuries to the chest wall should be considered in terms of the anatomy affected by the injury. Structures to be considered are ribs, lungs, heart, and mediastinal structures.

Never forget that the flow of oxygen into the lungs may be compromised at any point from the mouth or nostrils down to the alveoli, and so the assessment of the chest (as ever) begins with an assessment of the airway.

If the airway and cervical spine have been assessed and treated, move on to the neck and then the chest wall.

Laryngeal injury may accompany thoracic trauma, so make sure to assess the neck, especially if there is alteration of the player's voice, hoarseness, or stridor.

4.3.1 Assessment

Assess chest movement closely to ascertain the following:

- ✓ Respiratory rate
- ✓ Respiratory effort.
- ✓ Symmetry of chest movement:
  - Look for an obvious lack of movement on one side of the chest.
  - Look for an obvious flail segment. This is caused by fractures of three or more ribs and in two or more places in each of the affected ribs (this results in paradoxical breathing where the flail segment is pulled inward on inspiration and outward on exhalation).

Listen to the player in terms of both what they are saying and the respiratory noises they are making.

- Gurgling implies upper airway pathology.
- Stridor implies upper airway pathology.
- Coughing is a protective reflex and a positive sound.
- Wheezing implies lower respiratory tract pathology.

- Check trachea is central.
- Feel the neck for surgical emphysema.
- Feel the chest wall to assess pain or crepitus suggestive of a rib fracture.

It is unlikely that using a stethoscope will add anything to the initial pitchside assessment. If you suspect a pneumothorax is a possibility, then remove the player immediately and continue the assessment in the treatment room.

4.3.2 Traumatic Thoracic Conditions

Rib Fracture

In isolation, this requires analgesia and a 4- to 6-week recovery period. It is basically a diagnosis made after all life-threatening causes of chest injury have been excluded. The player will have palpable tenderness over the area, pain on inspiration, and possible crepitus examining the rib. They should not remain tachypnoeic, dyspnoeic, or tachycardic. If so, question whether or not you have the correct diagnosis. You must advise the player to seek further attention if they suddenly become short of breath, have increasing pain, or develop a productive cough. Treatment is analgesia.

Sternal Fracture

This is the result of a direct blow to the sternum. Tenderness over the sternum will be elicited along with anterior chest pain. The concern here is not directed toward the fracture, but rather the potential for an associated myocardial injury. An electrocardiogram is required, but if this is normal, an admission to hospital is unlikely to be necessary. Treatment is analgesia.

Flail Segment

This usually results in multiple rib fractures (three or more ribs fractured in two or more places). The chest wall fails to move, resulting in a paradoxical breathing pattern where the chest wall that is separate moves inward with inspiration. In association with underlying lung injury and poor respiratory effort caused by pain, this may result in hypoxia. Treatment is oxygen, analgesia, and immediate referral to hospital.

Pneumothorax

In a sporting context, this usually results from a fractured rib. Signs to look for are asymmetric chest wall expansion, hyperresonance on percussion or decreased air entry on auscultation. However, these signs may be very subtle and very difficult to pick up at pitchside. Presence of surgical emphysema in the neck, axilla, or around the chest wall is a far more specific finding in a patient with a pneumothorax. Differentiating between a rib fracture and a pneumothorax without hemodynamic compromise is made even harder when you take into account the fact that a player with a fracture will splint the affected side, resulting in "false-positive" clinical signs for pneumothorax.

If a player with a chest wall injury does not return to a normal breathing pattern within 5 minutes, a more significant injury should be assumed and the player removed from the field of play for serial assessments.

Treatment of a hemodynamically normal patient with a suspected pneumothorax is oxygen, analgesia, and referral to hospital.

Tension Pneumothorax

In this situation, the pneumothorax is associated with a one-way valve leak of air into the thoracic cavity with each breath taken by the patient. This results in a complete collapse of the lung and subsequent compression of the mediastinum. This in turn causes decrease in venous return to the heart and resulting hypotension and shock. The player will be critically unwell, with absent air entry in the affected lung, which may be hyper-resonant to percussion, and signs of shock (hypotension and tachycardia or they may be periarrest, at which point they will become bradycardic prior to losing their pulse). Neck veins may be dilated and the trachea deviated away from the affected side. The player will show marked respiratory distress.

Treatment of a player with a suspected tension pneumothorax (pneumothorax and shock) is to place a large bore intravenous (IV) cannula into the second intercostal space anteriorly in the midclavicular line. This is a **life-saving but temporizing** procedure that releases some of the pressure but converts the tension into a simple pneumothorax that will still require treatment with a chest drain.

Needle Decompression

Needle decompression is important to mention in this context as it is a life-saving yet relatively simple procedure to perform. However, it should not be undertaken unless the attending clinician is absolutely confident in their ability to have diagnosed the condition correctly.

Remember: the patient will be in extremis with this condition.

Ensure the player has 15 L of oxygen (O_2) via nonrebreather trauma mask.

- Identify the *second intercostal space* (between the second and the third ribs). This is best found by finding the angle of Louis, i.e., the manubriosternal joint, and moving directly laterally to the intercostal space at this level.
- Identify the *midclavicular line*—the midpoint between the sternoclavicular joint medially and the acromioclavicular joint laterally.
- Clean the skin with a sterile swab.
- Insert a 14- or 16-G IV cannula into the second IC space in the midclavicular line aiming to enter the space just above the third rib to avoid the neurovascular bundle.

- Advance the cannula into the space and remove the needle leaving the plastic cannula in situ. On removal of the needle, a hiss of air should be apparent and the player's condition should improve quickly as they ventilate.
- Secure the cannula with tape and transfer to hospital.

Differential Diagnoses of Tension Pneumothorax

You should consider massive hemothorax of the chest, where blood accumulates in the pleural cavity rather than air. In this case, a player will also be hypotensive and tachycardic with decreased air entry and respiratory distress.

Diaphragmatic rupture is very uncommon but may also cause similar symptoms of respiratory distress and hemodynamic compromise associated with decreased air entry into the affected side.

4.4 Abdominal Trauma

Evaluation of the abdomen (and pelvis) should take place once an ABC assessment has been made. This occurs as part of the assessment of circulation and as such, the player's vital signs of pulse and blood pressure should be taken (if not done already).

Remember that lower chest wall injuries are also associated with upper abdominal injuries. In anyone who you think may have a fracture of the lower ribs (10–12), you should have a high index of suspicion that they may also have an associated intra-abdominal injury.

4.4.1 Anatomy

The abdomen is vulnerable because it contains both solid and hollow viscous organs in addition to major vascular structures. In football, blunt trauma is responsible for the vast majority of injuries, with the abdominal musculature responsible for protecting the underlying structures.

It should be remembered that the actual abdominal cavity varies with respiration and can rise as far as the fourth intercostal space during expiration. Depending on the state of respiration, the solid organs of the liver and spleen can become more exposed, increasing the risk of injury. Hollow viscous organs tend to be injured in penetrating or sudden deceleration trauma, and as such in football this rarely occurs.

The abdomen can be divided into quadrants:

- *Right upper quadrant:* liver, gallbladder, pancreas, duodenum, ascending colon, transverse colon, right kidney and ureter, hepatic flexure, right adrenal.
- *Left upper quadrant:* stomach, spleen, transverse colon, splenic flexure, descending colon, pancreas, left kidney and ureter, left adrenal.
- *Right iliac fossa:* caecum, appendix, ascending colon, right ovary.
- *Left iliac fossa:* descending colon, sigmoid colon, left ovary.

Other structures found in the midline include the aorta and inferior vena cava, the bladder, and the uterus

4.4.2 Assessment

Initial assessment should follow the framework described in Chapter 1.

Do not be distracted from assessing the airway, cervical spine, and breathing prior to assessing the abdomen as part of circulation. Consider the proximity of the chest and abdominal cavities, and ensure a thorough respiratory examination even if the only complaint is of abdominal pain.

Signs of shock after abdominal trauma (tachycardia, narrowed pulse pressure, hypotension) mandate emergency transfer to hospital with ongoing fluid resuscitation. Surgical intervention will be required if a sustained response is not achieved.

Distinguishing the actual cause of abdominal pain is secondary to ensuring that the player has received analgesia, IV access has been obtained and fluids have been started where available, and transfer to a center for definitive care has been organized.

In the hemodynamically normal player, findings suggestive of significant injury again necessitate transfer for further management. Remember the importance of repeated assessments to detect any delayed onset of bleeding or peritonitis resulting in changes in the clinical picture.

Look for signs of the following:

- ✓ Bruising.
- ✓ Abdominal distension.
- ✓ Absence of normal abdominal movement with respiration **suggesting splinting of the abdomen.**

Listen for the presence or absence of bowel sounds.

- Palpate tenderness including rebound.
- Assess for guarding and also pain referred to the back or shoulder suggesting diaphragmatic irritation from leaking blood.

4.4.3 Trauma

Trauma can be either blunt or penetrating.

Blunt. Blunt injury is much more common in sport than penetrating injury. It causes direct trauma to a solid organ such as the liver, kidney, or spleen, resulting in bleeding or rupture of the organ. A direct kick to the abdomen can deliver enough force to cause such an injury, and certain medical conditions such as glandular fever can increase the likelihood of splenic injury, due to the increased size of the organ that is an inherent part of this condition.

Hollow viscera such as duodenum can be injured by sudden deceleration forces that cause these mobile structures to tear at the points where they are fixed. These types of injury are rare in football but may occur in collisions at speed such as running into the goal post.

Penetrating. These types of injuries are very rare in sport generally and do not readily occur in football. A kick to the abdomen with the studs facing up may cause a penetrating wound, but due to the size of studs commonly used in football, it is exceptionally rare that this will actually result in an intra-abdominal injury.

Specific Traumatic Injuries

Spleen

The spleen is found in the left upper quadrant and is vulnerable to direct trauma, especially if swollen as a result of medical conditions such as infectious mononucleosis or leukemia. In its normal state, it is about the size of a clenched fist and lies just below the diaphragm, with some protection afforded by the left lower ribs 9–12. Direct trauma can result in capsular hematomas which may bleed at variable rates. Depending on the extent of the injury, the player may suddenly collapse if blood loss occurs quickly, though classically it may take time before there is any deterioration in the clinical picture. This type of injury can result in left shoulder tip pain due to diaphragmatic irritation from the bleeding.

Initial management is to provide oxygen, analgesia, and fluid resuscitation as required. Imaging such as ultrasound can be useful to diagnose free fluid in the abdominal cavity, but CT is the best option if available. Many injuries can be managed conservatively, but a splenectomy may be required in more serious cases.

Liver

The liver lies in the right upper quadrant and is also vulnerable to direct trauma, especially from a kick to this area. It is protected by the right ribs 9–12 but may be more vulnerable to trauma in conditions such as alcohol hepatitis, viral hepatitis, infectious mononucleosis, or leukemia. The liver extends further into the abdominal cavity during deep inspiration. Lacerations to the liver are exceptionally rare in football, though subcapsular hematomas can occur after a direct blow to the right upper quadrant. If you suspect such an injury, oxygenate, administer analgesia, and transfer the player for further management and CT imaging.

Diaphragm

The diaphragm is a muscular structure that separates the chest from the abdominal cavity. It is prone to injury in significant blunt abdominal force such as a kick. This force can cause it to rupture, something that occurs more commonly on the left side because the right is protected by the liver. Rupture may cause abdominal contents to herniate into the chest cavity, compressing and collapsing the left lung. Clinical signs in this case will be of decreased air entry into the left chest and may be associated with shock. These signs may be similar to those of a tension pneumothorax. Management involves providing the player with oxygen and analgesia, with urgent transfer.

If there is doubt as to whether the player has a tension pneumothorax or a ruptured diaphragm with herniation, treat for the former, as this is more common and the management of needle decompression is life-saving.

Bowel

Large and small bowel injury is rare in football, but case reports have described both. Significant blunt force can cause rupture of the bowel from tears that occur at the sites where the bowel is fixed. Symptoms may be delayed depending on the size of the tear and the onset of peritonitis. The retroperitoneal position of the duodenum can mean that signs are difficult to detect clinically, so a high index of suspicion should be employed in any player who has sustained a significant mechanism of injury but appears to be well initially. Lumbar spine fractures have been described in association with injuries to the colon. As above, **initial management is to provide oxygen, analgesia, and fluid resuscitation as required,** with urgent transfer for operative management in the vast majority of cases.

Genitourinary

These can be subdivided into upper and lower urological injuries where the vast majority of lower and genital injuries can be avoided with the use of protective cups.

The kidneys are protected by the lower ribs 10–12 as well as the psoas muscles. They are still vulnerable to direct blunt trauma that compresses them against the lumbar spine resulting in renal contusions. The player may complain of increasing flank pain and there may be associated flank bruising. Urinalysis may show microscopic hematuria, which is usually managed conservatively as long as the player's vital signs remain unaffected. Evidence of gross hematuria or symptoms of shock mandate immediate referral for investigation. Obviously in the case of shock, the player will need a full ABC assessment and resuscitation.

Rectus Abdominis

The paired rectus abdominis muscles run from the xiphoid process and the fifth to seventh costal cartilages down to the pubic symphysis. The most common rectus injury is a muscular strain, but occasionally a rectus hematoma can occur as the result of direct trauma. The hematoma arises from injury to the superior or inferior epigastric vessels. The most common presentation is with abdominal pain which may be sudden or develop over a few hours. A fever may occur in association with other nonspecific findings such as anorexia or vomiting. A palpable mass may be present which may help to distinguish the diagnosis from other causes of abdominal pain. There is a risk of mortality from the condition in cases where there is hypovolemic shock from blood loss.

Management is dependent on the extent of blood loss and symptoms, with operative intervention being required in cases where there is hypovolemia. Otherwise, analgesia, rest, and ice are usually all that is required.

4.5 Pelvic Trauma

The pelvis should be assessed as part of circulation once the airway, cervical spine, and breathing assessments have been carried out.

Pelvic injury is very common in sport and especially football, where strains to the soft tissues that support the pelvis are common. Life-threatening injuries are rare in football but must be looked for and dealt with quickly to minimize the risk to life.

Remember that hip and back pain may be referred to the knee and this can be a compounding factor when making an assessment.

As with the abdomen, the pelvic cavity houses many organs that may themselves be responsible for life-threatening nontraumatic causes of pain, such as a ruptured ectopic pregnancy. You could save a player's life by being able to adequately resuscitate them from such conditions using oxygen, IV fluids, and analgesics while you arrange transfer for definitive treatment.

4.5.1 Anatomy

The pelvis is a large, ring-like structure that comprises the sacrum posteriorly, with the coccyx inferior to it. These link to the ilia on either side via the sacroiliac joints. The ischium and pubis complete the ring anteriorly, joining on either side at the pubis symphysis. A number of strong ligaments help to support the pelvis and create a much more stable girdle than seen in the shoulder, for example. This girdle helps to transmit the forces required to enable movement of the lower limbs while supporting the rest of the upper body. Of importance within the pelvis are the bowel, bladder, ureters, iliac vessels, and reproductive organs—all of which can be damaged by blunt or penetrating trauma. The hip joint comprises the femoral head as the ball within the acetabular socket. The acetabulum is formed by the meeting of the ilium, ischium, and pubis. Movement at the hip joint is multidirectional, so knowledge of the muscles responsible for these movements is helpful in determining soft-tissue causes of pain (**Table 4.3**).

4.5.2 Assessment

Given the potentially catastrophic outcome of a pelvic fracture, an adequate assessment of the airway, cervical spine, and breathing must be made before turning your attention to the pelvis as part of circulation. A catastrophic pelvic fracture is unlikely in football. However, in the case of a player who has landed from a height directly onto their hip or pelvis, there should be no doubt that there is the potential for life-threatening hemorrhage from pelvic injury. Be aware of the mechanism of injury and if you do not see the event itself, then get as much information as possible from those who may have witnessed it.

Having assessed and treated airway and breathing, assess the pelvis as part of your circulatory assessment. Check pulse and BP.

Table 4.3

Muscles associated with hip movements

Type of movement	Muscles
Flexion	Sartorius, rectus femoris, and iliopsoas
Extension	Gluteus maximus and hamstring muscles (semimembranosus, semitendinosis, and biceps femoris
Adduction	Gracilis, pectineus, and the three adductor muscles (longus, brevis, and magnus)
Abduction	Gluteus medius and minimus and tensor fascia lata
External rotation	Piriformis, gluteus minimus, obturator internus, and quadratus femoris
Internal rotation	Gluteus medius, adductor magnus, semimembranosus, and semitendinosis

4

- ✓ Obvious deformity/asymmetry? How is the player holding their leg?
- ✓ (Remember that the source of pain may be referred and examine the joints above and below the one you think is injured. In the case of the pelvis, for example, pay attention to the lumbosacral spine and the knee as well as the pelvis and hip.)
- ✓ Bruising or bleeding?
- ✓ Swelling?

- **Do not spring the pelvis**—This is only likely to worsen any bleeding and possibly convert a stable pelvic fracture into an unstable one.
- Palpate the iliac crests from posterior to anterior starting at the sacroiliac joint if possible and moving anteriorly. Assess for groin tenderness, then palpate the hips starting at the greater trochanter and again moving anteriorly.
- Assess for tenderness, swelling, or crepitus.

- If any movement of the pelvis is to be made (other than as part of a logroll), it should involve a movement, effectively closing the pelvis rather than springing it backward and forcing the pelvis open. This is done by holding the iliac crests and gently pulling them anteromedially.
- Movement of the hips should be done in the order of active first and passive second, with due note being made of the range of movement and the directions that elicit pain. Ensure you examine the femur and knee joints as well.

4.5.3 Fractures

Pelvic Ring Fractures

Fractures involving the pelvic ring are usually associated with blunt high-energy trauma and are therefore rare in football. However, disruption of the ring results in bleeding into a large potential space in the form of the pelvic cavity. Up to 4 L of blood can accumulate within the pelvis and the retroperitoneal space, so shock and life-threatening hemorrhage can easily occur in any unstable fracture. Irrespective of the mechanism of injury, in the first instance the management is exactly the same.

Complications of pelvic fractures are usually related to the associated blood loss, which can be markedly worsened if the injury is compound. Stopping ongoing blood loss involves splinting the player's pelvis using a readily available pelvic binder, or even a large towel or sheet. Other problems such as associated spine trauma should be assumed and sought for in addition to injury to the pelvic organs themselves.

Management is based on the primary assessment described in Chapter 1.

- Assess ABC with the pelvis being assessed as part of circulation.
- Do not forget to consider the cervical spine—a pelvic injury is a significant distracting injury and as such a cervical collar is a sensible precautionary measure.
- Remember **not** to spring the pelvis as this may worsen bleeding.

Using a pelvic binder or a sheet tied around the hips may help reduce a fracture and minimize ongoing blood loss.

Simple measures such as oxygenation, IV analgesia, and fluids are useful measures while you arrange transfer to the nearest emergency department.

Dislocation of the Hip

Dislocation of the hip involves considerable force and tends to occur as a result of high-energy trauma. Although uncommon in football, these injuries do occur and can be seen with or without the presence of an associated fracture of either the femoral neck or the acetabulum. Uneven surfaces with awkward landings from jumps have been suggested as potential reasons for this type of injury occurring in the absence of the high-energy trauma we would usually expect to see.

The player will complain of excruciating pain in the affected side and there will be shortening of the affected leg with a variable appearance to the hip depending on whether the dislocation is anterior or posterior. Approximately 90% of hip dislocations are posterior and the player is likely to have their hip flexed, adducted, and internally rotated. The sciatic nerve may be involved and a neurovascular assessment should be made.

Management involves assessing for other injuries, oxygenating, providing analgesia, splinting, and transferring to hospital for definitive management, usually involving reduction in theater.

Avulsion Fractures

This type of fracture is much more common in adolescents than in adults. It is caused by a sudden violent contraction, which can be either eccentric or concentric, resulting in the muscle pulling off its bony attachment.

In football, striking the ball involves hip flexion and knee extension achieved through contraction of rectus femoris and this can result in an avulsion at its origin from the anterior inferior iliac spine. Pain is usually sudden, with palpable tenderness at the site as well as pain on initiating hip flexion. Avulsions of the insertion of the hamstrings at the ischial tuberosity can also occur when sprinting. This results in pain on knee flexion as well as palpable tenderness over the ischial tuberosity. Avulsion of the sartorius occurs at its insertion at the anterior superior iliac spine. This tends to be caused by the explosive hip flexion required when jumping, and results in pain over the muscle insertion as well as pain when actively flexing the hip.

Management of all avulsion fractures is similar and involves protected weight bearing, ice, and analgesia. X-ray confirms the diagnosis in the majority of cases. Depending on fragment size, referral may be required for orthopaedic fixation.

Stress Fractures

Stress fractures usually affect either the femoral neck or the pubic ramus. Pathology is of force transfer from weakened muscles that cannot cope with the loads to which they are subjected, and this stress is transferred to the bone which sustains repetitive microtrauma and fractures. This is more likely to occur when there has been a rapid increase in training schedules or a change to the surface on which the player is training.

In a femoral neck fracture, the player usually complains of pain affecting the front of the groin which worsens during activity but settles with periods of rest. There may be tenderness palpating the inguinal area, with pain on hip rotation. Players with a pubic ramus fracture may also complain of pain in the anterior groin but with tenderness present on palpation of the pubic ramus.

The diagnosis can be very difficult to make especially if the X-rays are normal, so a high degree of suspicion should be maintained in someone whose symptoms do not settle. Further imaging may be required.

4.6 Limb Trauma

Limb injuries, while unlikely to cause mortality, are the biggest cause of morbidity faced by footballers. Many injuries will be the result of overuse resulting in problems such as stress fractures. The underlying etiology of these injuries differs from those that occur as a result of trauma and this needs to be taken into account when deciding the best course of management for any particular injury.

Clinical assessment of the injury using the traditional look, feel, move method will probably allow most conditions to be correctly identified. Remember to always assess the joint above and below the site of the injury, and if in doubt, further assessment and radiological examination will be necessary at the nearest emergency department. In most cases, simply splinting appropriately and administering analgesia will be sufficient in the immediate period after the injury.

Compound Injuries. Particular issues will be caused by the association of a wound with a fracture. You must assume that the wound and fracture have an anatomical connection and that the player therefore has a compound fracture. In most cases, this will require formal exploration and the wound to be washed out in theater. Similarly, any wound overlying a joint should be assumed to have penetrated the joint capsule. Do not close these wounds unless you are absolutely comfortable that you have seen the wound in its entirety and that the joint is unaffected. In these situations, clean the wound as best you can, cover with a saline-soaked gauze swab, bandage the wound with the limb in a neutral position, and then rest in sling or box splint. Transfer to the nearest emergency department.

Dislocation or Fracture? In many situations, the clinical diagnosis will be apparent due to the classic appearance of the injury. For example in the case of an anterior shoulder dislocation the classic clinical appearance is of a squared-off deformity at the acromion with loss of the normal curvature of the humeral head as it sits inferiorly to the glenoid. This clinical appearance is unlikely to be confused with an isolated fracture of the humerus; however, on occasion there will be an associated fracture of the greater tuberosity related to the dislocation and you should bear this in mind before any reduction of the shoulder is undertaken prior to imaging taking place.

In any situation where there is either a fracture or a dislocation resulting in clinical signs of neurovascular compromise distal to the injury the immediate management should involve analgesia and immediate reduction of the fracture and/or dislocation **without** waiting for radiographic confirmation. This type of situation is classically seen in fracture dislocations of the ankle.

4.6.1 Upper Limb

Shoulder

Clavicle

This is a relatively common injury in football, from either a fall onto an outstretched hand or direct trauma. Examination will reveal localized tenderness over the fracture site with or without a visible deformity depending on displacement of the fracture. Initial treatment is with a sling.

Acromioclavicular Dislocation

This can occur in isolation or in association with a fracture. The dislocation can be graded depending on the ligaments involved. Usually the management is conservative. Initial treatment is with a sling.

Sternoclavicular Joint Dislocation

Sternoclavicular joint dislocation usually occurs anteriorly resulting in pain and deformity of the sternoclavicular joint on the affected side. A palpable firm tender swelling is noted at the junction of the sternum and clavicle. Examination should look for associated injuries underlying this such as pneumothorax. Treatment is analgesia and sling. The majority need no further treatment and functional recovery is good without operative intervention. The athlete should be informed there will however be a residual cosmetically noticeable swelling.

Posterior sternoclavicular joint dislocations are exceptionally rare but are an emergency when they do occur. The posterior displacement of the clavicle can cause compression of the underlying vessels especially the brachiocephalic vein impeding blood flow. The symptoms may take a few hours or even days to fully develop and diagnosis can be difficult to make with plain imaging. CT will enable the diagnosis to be made. Reduction is required and given the inherent instability of the clavicle operative open fixation is usually required. If symptoms of shock or limb ischaemia are noted then the clavicle can attempt to be pulled forward although this can be exceptionally difficult to achieve, even in a theatre environment.

Neck of Humerus Fracture

This is an unusual injury in sport. When it occurs, it is usually due to a fall onto the outstretched hand with or without a further load landing on top of the player (e.g., another player). The normal contour of the shoulder is unlikely to be lost, thus distinguishing it from a dislocation. There may, however, be significant swelling associated. Ensure no neurovascular complications and place in a sling.

Dislocated Shoulder

The vast majority will dislocate anteriorly resulting in loss of the normal curvature of the shoulder as the humeral head lies anteroinferiorly to the glenoid. Treatment is with analgesia with or without sedation followed by reduction.

A balance needs to be struck as to where and when to reduce. There are a number of different aspects that need to be considered. Without imaging, there is the possibility of an associated fracture being missed. In real terms, the most common type of fracture that occurs with shoulder dislocations is an avulsion of the greater tuberosity. This will not usually result in any change in managing the reduction, so it could be argued that it is best to just proceed and achieve the reduction at pitchside. The risk of this, however, is twofold. First, if, after the reduction, subsequent X-rays are taken and they reveal there has been a fracture, it could be argued that this was the result of the technique used to achieve the reduction rather than a consequence of the initial injury. This raises a number of medicolegal issues.

Second and more importantly, there may be an associated fracture that is in fact either impinging on the joint or affecting the humeral shaft. The reduction of these injuries would be better undertaken in hospital and possibly in theatre. Without an initial X-ray, it can be difficult to exclude these issues.

Taking into account the problems mentioned above, there are probably three situations where it may be sensible to proceed directly to reduction:

- In someone who has a previous history of dislocations—these players will also probably know the best technique to use to achieve their reduction.
- In someone with associated distal neurovascular compromise (highly unusual in an isolated dislocation).
- In someone for whom there will be a significant delay in transfer to the nearest emergency department.

In players with significant swelling or if there is any doubt as to the diagnosis, splint the arm in a sling and transfer for imaging.

Reduction Techniques. You will not be able to reduce a dislocation if the player is not relaxed. Analgesia will be required. Entonox is ideal if available.

There are three simple techniques to try that all avoid the potential problems of "forcing" the head into the joint, and the associated risks of causing fractures by doing so.

- **Have the player lie supine.** Supporting the affected arm, gently lift it in an upward direction trying to achieve forward flexion of about 90 degrees at the shoulder. If you can continue to support the arm and gently pull it upward toward the sky, the player's body weight will act as traction. Holding this position, the shoulder will reduce as the muscles relax, allowing the dislocation to reduce.
- **Have the player lie semirecumbently.** Extend the elbow and apply gentle traction to pull the arm in a downward direction, i.e., toward the player's feet. This will have the effect of disengaging the dislocation inferiorly, allowing reduction. All that is required of the operator is to lean backward while holding the player's arm. No other force is required.

- **Have the player lie prone**, with their arm hanging over the side of the treatment table. Ask them to hold onto a weight such as a water bottle. Gravity will again allow the dislocation to reduce.

All of these techniques are relatively safe to perform as they avoid forcing the joint. They also all share the same principles of being performed **gently** and **gradually.**

Elbow

Dislocated Elbow

This may or may not be associated with fracture. The appearance will be of loss of the normal anatomical triangle formed between the olecranon and the epicondyles on either side. A visible deformity will be apparent. A check must be made for the presence or loss of pulses. If pulses are absent, then immediate reduction should be considered unless there is rapid access to the nearest emergency department.

Most dislocations occur in a posterolateral direction. Reduction is achieved by flexing the elbow. With a second person applying traction distally, use your thumbs to push the olecranon in a distal direction. Once reduced, the normal "triangle" appearances will be seen. Emergency department assessment will be required in all cases and admission may be required in some.

Radial Head Fracture

This is a relatively common injury as a result of a fall onto the outstretched hand. An effusion will be seen with tenderness over the radial head on palpation. Treatment is a sling and usually conservative management.

Olecranon Fracture

This is an uncommon injury that occurs from landing on the point of the elbow. Pull of triceps may cause separation of the fracture and make operative treatment necessary. Sling and transfer for imaging.

Supracondylar Fracture

This is more common in children but can be associated with neurovascular complications. Sling and transfer for imaging.

Wrist

Distal Radius and/or Ulna Fracture

This is a very common injury from falling onto the outstretched hand. Pain, swelling, bruising, and deformity may be evident. Any obvious clinical deformity will invariably mean that the player will require manipulation of the fracture, so splint, administer analgesia, and refer to the emergency department. It is exceptionally unlikely that a wrist injury would ever need to be "pulled" at pitchside due to neurovascular compromise.

Scaphoid Fracture

This is a relatively common injury and a very common cause of litigation due to missed or maltreated injuries. In any wrist injury, assess for tenderness over the anatomical snuffbox. Swelling is common in this area. Assess for pain over the snuffbox when telescoping the thumb or index finger.

Thumb

Bennett's Fracture Dislocation

Direct trauma to the thumb may result in a fracture dislocation of the thumb carpometacarpal joint. This will require reduction and/or fixation, so splint and immediately transfer anyone with a deformity affecting the thumb.

Ulnar Collateral Thumb Disruption

This occurs due to hyperabduction of the thumb. Stability of the thumb must be assessed and ulnar collateral ligament integrity documented.

Other Injuries

Beware of any rotational deformity in finger injuries. These are far more common in phalangeal fractures than in metacarpal fractures (which tend to do well with conservative management). Rotational deformity is exceptionally debilitating and may be a career-threatening injury, so refer such cases to the emergency department.

4.6.2 Lower Limb

The main problem with diagnosing an acute lower limb injury is that, in order to assess function, you may need to make the decision to try to stand the player up. Only do this in a graded fashion after making your look, feel, move assessment.

In many cases, especially the conditions documented below, it will be obvious that there is a significant injury, so there will be no issue in trying to move the player. If, however, there is any doubt as to the severity of the injury, do not attempt to get the player to walk until you have stretchered them from the field and made a more comprehensive assessment at pitchside.

Femoral Shaft Fracture

This injury is potentially life-threatening, especially if compound. It is the result of significant traumatic forces, and as such is relatively uncommon in football. The management is entirely based around the ABC approach with the airway and cervical spine taking priority.

IV access should be established as soon as possible to allow the administration of IV morphine as well as fluid resuscitation if needed. Significant blood may be lost from the fracture site and shock may become evident especially if the fracture is compound. Analgesia is best provided by a femoral nerve block (see Section 5.1 in Chapter 5) and this may allow you to move the player as well as splint the limb. Do not worry about the risk of "masking" the symptoms of a compartment syndrome—the primary aim initially is to resuscitate and administer analgesia.

Knee Injuries

If an effusion is present at the pitchside, the player has sustained either a cruciate ligament injury or a fracture. Both of these conditions will result in blood in the joint. Stretcher the player from the pitch and do not allow them to try to walk. Administer analgesia, splint, and transfer for further management.

Patella Dislocation

This is a relatively common injury that can be easily treated. In many players, these will be recurrent. The majority dislocate laterally and it will reduce if you extend the knee while applying gentle pressure to the patella in a medial direction. Entonox is an ideal agent if this is available to facilitate the procedure.

Tibial Shaft Fracture

This again is a relatively common injury in many contact sports. Initial management involves assessment of distal neurovascular compromise, analgesia, and splinting the limb prior to transfer.

Ankle Fracture Dislocation

This is a musculoskeletal emergency that will necessitate immediate reduction if there is a threat of either the skin breaking down from bony pressure or neurovascular compromise. This is one of the most likely injuries to be associated with vascular compromise due to the displacement of the anatomy.

Most fracture dislocations will result in the ankle mortice being disrupted with the talus shifted in a posterior direction.

With an assistant applying countertraction, ensure the knee is in a flexed position to allow muscle relaxation. Holding the heel, apply gentle traction in an inferior direction to allow disimpaction of the fracture first before correcting any medial or lateral disruption. There will be a notable clunk as the dislocation reduces. Recheck pulses and ensure the foot "pinks up." Remember that the injury may still be unstable, so splinting will be required next. Continue to observe the pulses and ensure the ankle stays in joint.

If the injury is compound, proceed as described above. Take a picture of the wound if you can, then clean with saline-soaked swabs. Leave a clean saline swab over the wound before splinting.

References

[1] McCrory P, Meeuwisse W, Johnston K, et al. Consensus Statement on Concussion in Sport: the 3rd International Conference on Concussion in Sport held in Zurich, November 2008. Br J Sports Med. 2009; 43 Suppl 1:i76–i90

[2] SCAT3. SCAT3. Br J Sports Med. 2013; 47(5):259

[3] Scottish Intercollegiate Guidelines Network (SIGN). Guideline 110: early management of patients with a head injury. http://www.sign.ac.uk/guidelines/fulltext/110/

SCAT3™

FIFA®

Sport Concussion Assessment Tool – 3rd Edition

For use by medical professionals only

Name

Date/Time of Injury
Date of Assessment

Examiner

What is the SCAT3?[1]

The SCAT3 is a standardized tool for evaluating injured athletes for concussion and can be used in athletes aged from 13 years and older. It supersedes the original SCAT and the SCAT2 published in 2005 and 2009, respectively. For younger persons, ages 12 and under, please use the Child SCAT3. The SCAT3 is designed for use by medical professionals. If you are not qualified, please use the Sport Concussion Recognition Tool. Preseason baseline testing with the SCAT3 can be helpful for interpreting post-injury test scores.

Specific instructions for use of the SCAT3 are provided on page 3. If you are not familiar with the SCAT3, please read through these instructions carefully. This tool may be freely copied in its current form for distribution to individuals, teams, groups and organizations. Any revision or any reproduction in a digital form requires approval by the Concussion in Sport Group.

NOTE: The diagnosis of a concussion is a clinical judgment, ideally made by a medical professional. The SCAT3 should not be used solely to make, or exclude, the diagnosis of concussion in the absence of clinical judgement. An athlete may have a concussion even if their SCAT3 is "normal".

What is a concussion?

A concussion is a disturbance in brain function caused by a direct or indirect force to the head. It results in a variety of non-specific signs and/or symptoms (some examples listed below) and most often does not involve loss of consciousness. Concussion should be suspected in the presence of **any one or more** of the following:

- Symptoms (e.g., headache), or
- Physical signs (e.g., unsteadiness), or
- Impaired brain function (e.g. confusion) or
- Abnormal behaviour (e.g., change in personality).

SIDELINE ASSESSMENT

Indications for Emergency Management

NOTE: A hit to the head can sometimes be associated with a more serious brain injury. Any of the following warrants consideration of activating emergency procedures and urgent transportation to the nearest hospital:

- Glasgow Coma score less than 15
- Deteriorating mental status
- Potential spinal injury
- Progressive, worsening symptoms or new neurologic signs

Potential signs of concussion?

If any of the following signs are observed after a direct or indirect blow to the head, the athlete should stop participation, be evaluated by a medical professional and **should not be permitted to return to sport the same day** if a concussion is suspected.

Any loss of consciousness?	Y	N
"If so, how long?"		
Balance or motor incoordination (stumbles, slow/laboured movements, etc.)?	Y	N
Disorientation or confusion (inability to respond appropriately to questions)?	Y	N
Loss of memory:	Y	N
"If so, how long?"		
"Before or after the injury?"		
Blank or vacant look:	Y	N
Visible facial injury in combination with any of the above:	Y	N

1 Glasgow coma scale (GCS)

Best eye response (E)	
No eye opening	1
Eye opening in response to pain	2
Eye opening to speech	3
Eyes opening spontaneously	4
Best verbal response (V)	
No verbal response	1
Incomprehensible sounds	2
Inappropriate words	3
Confused	4
Oriented	5
Best motor response (M)	
No motor response	1
Extension to pain	2
Abnormal flexion to pain	3
Flexion/Withdrawal to pain	4
Localizes to pain	5
Obeys commands	6
Glasgow Coma score (E + V + M)	of 15

GCS should be recorded for all athletes in case of subsequent deterioration.

2 Maddocks Score[3]

"I am going to ask you a few questions, please listen carefully and give your best effort."

Modified Maddocks questions (1 point for each correct answer)

What venue are we at today?	0	1
Which half is it now?	0	1
Who scored last in this match?	0	1
What team did you play last week/game?	0	1
Did your team win the last game?	0	1
Maddocks score		of 5

Maddocks score is validated for sideline diagnosis of concussion only and is not used for serial testing.

Notes: Mechanism of Injury ("tell me what happened"?):

Any athlete with a suspected concussion should be REMOVED FROM PLAY, medically assessed, monitored for deterioration (i.e., should not be left alone) and should not drive a motor vehicle until cleared to do so by a medical professional. No athlete diagnosed with concussion should be returned to sports participation on the day of Injury.

SCAT3 SPORT CONCUSSION ASSESMENT TOOL 3 | **PAGE 1**

2[illegible]9

Appendix I Sport Concussion Assessment Tool 3 (SCAT 3).[2]

BACKGROUND

Name: Date:
Examiner:
Sport/team/school: Date/time of injury:
Age: Gender: M F
Years of education completed:
Dominant hand: right left neither
How many concussions do you think you have had in the past?
When was the most recent concussion?
How long was your recovery from the most recent concussion?
Have you ever been hospitalized or had medical imaging done for a head injury? Y N
Have you ever been diagnosed with headaches or migraines? Y N
Do you have a learning disability, dyslexia, ADD/ADHD? Y N
Have you ever been diagnosed with depression, anxiety or other psychiatric disorder? Y N
Has anyone in your family ever been diagnosed with any of these problems? Y N
Are you on any medications? If yes, please list: Y N

SCAT3 to be done in resting state. Best done 10 or more minutes post excercise.

SYMPTOM EVALUATION

3 How do you feel?

"You should score yourself on the following symptoms, based on how you feel now"

	none	mild		moderate		severe	
Headache	0	1	2	3	4	5	6
"Pressure in head"	0	1	2	3	4	5	6
Neck Pain	0	1	2	3	4	5	6
Nausea or vomiting	0	1	2	3	4	5	6
Dizziness	0	1	2	3	4	5	6
Blurred vision	0	1	2	3	4	5	6
Balance problems	0	1	2	3	4	5	6
Sensitivity to light	0	1	2	3	4	5	6
Sensitivity to noise	0	1	2	3	4	5	6
Feeling slowed down	0	1	2	3	4	5	6
Feeling like "in a fog"	0	1	2	3	4	5	6
"Don't feel right"	0	1	2	3	4	5	6
Difficulty concentrating	0	1	2	3	4	5	6
Difficulty remembering	0	1	2	3	4	5	6
Fatigue or low energy	0	1	2	3	4	5	6
Confusion	0	1	2	3	4	5	6
Drowsiness	0	1	2	3	4	5	6
Trouble falling asleep	0	1	2	3	4	5	6
More emotional	0	1	2	3	4	5	6
Irritability	0	1	2	3	4	5	6
Sadness	0	1	2	3	4	5	6
Nervous or Anxious	0	1	2	3	4	5	6

Total number of symptoms (Maximum possible 22)
Symptom severity score (Maximum possible 132)

Do the symptoms get worse with physical activity? Y N
Do the symptoms get worse with mental activity? Y N

self rated / self rated and clinician monitored
clinician interview / self rated with parent input

Overall rating: If you know the athlete well prior to the injury, how different is the athlete acting compared to his/her usual self?

Please circle one response

no different	very different	unsure	N/A

Scoring on the SCAT3 should not be used as a stand-alone method to diagnose concussion, measure recovery or make decisions about an athlete's readiness to return to competition after concussion. Since signs and symptoms may evolve over time, it is important to consider repeat evaluation in the acute assessment of concussion.

COGNITIVE & PHYSICAL EVALUATION

4 Cognitive assessment

Standardized Assessment of Concussion (SAC)[4]

Orientation (1 point for each correct answer)

What month is it?	0	1
What is the date today?	0	1
What is the day of the week?	0	1
What year is it?	0	1
What time is it right now? (within 1 hour)	0	1
Orientation score		of 5

Immediate memory

List	Trial 1		Trial 2		Trial 3		Alternative word list		
elbow	0	1	0	1	0	1	candle	baby	finger
apple	0	1	0	1	0	1	paper	monkey	penny
carpet	0	1	0	1	0	1	sugar	perfume	blanket
saddle	0	1	0	1	0	1	sandwich	sunset	lemon
bubble	0	1	0	1	0	1	wagon	iron	insect
Total									

Immediate memory score total of 15

Concentration: Digits Backward

List	Trial 1		Alternative digit list		
4-9-3	0	1	6-2-9	5-2-6	4-1-5
3-8-1-4	0	1	3-2-7-9	1-7-9-5	4-9-6-8
6-2-9-7-1	0	1	1-5-2-8-6	3-8-5-2-7	6-1-8-4-3
7-1-8-4-6-2	0	1	5-3-9-1-4-8	8-3-1-9-6-4	7-2-4-8-5-6
Total of 4					

Concentration: Month in Reverse Order (1 pt. for entire sequence correct)

Dec-Nov-Oct-Sept-Aug-Jul-Jun-May-Apr-Mar-Feb-Jan 0 1

Concentration score of 5

5 Neck Examination:

Range of motion Tenderness Upper and lower limb sensation & strength

Findings:

6 Balance examination

Do one or both of the following tests.

Footwear (shoes, barefoot, braces, tape, etc.)

Modified Balance Error Scoring System (BESS) testing[5]

Which foot was tested (i.e. which is the **non-dominant** foot) Left Right

Testing surface (hard floor, field, etc.)

Condition

Double leg stance: Errors
Single leg stance (non-dominant foot): Errors
Tandem stance (non-dominant foot at back): Errors

And /Or

Tandem gait[6,7]

Time (best of 4 trials): seconds

7 Coordination examination

Upper limb coordination

Which arm was tested Left Right

Coordination score of 1

8 SAC Delayed Recall[4]

Delayed recall score of 5

Appendix I Sport Concussion Assessment Tool 3 (SCAT 3).[2]

INSTRUCTIONS

Words in *italics* throughout the SCAT3 are the instructions given to the athlete by the tester.

Symptom Scale

"You should score yourself on the following symptoms, based on how you feel now".

To be completed by the athlete. In situations where the symptom scale is being completed after exercise, it should still be done in a resting state, at least 10 minutes post exercise.

For total number of symptoms, maximum possible is 22.

For Symptom severity score, add all scores in table, maximum possible is 22×6 = 132.

SAC[4]

Immediate Memory

"I am going to test your memory. I will read you a list of words and when I am done, repeat back as many words as you can remember, in any order."

Trials 2 & 3:

"I am going to repeat the same list again. Repeat back as many words as you can remember in any order, even if you said the word before."

Complete all 3 trials regardless of score on trial 1 & 2. Read the words at a rate of one per second. **Score 1 pt. for each correct response.** Total score equals sum across all 3 trials. Do not inform the athlete that delayed recall will be tested.

Concentration

Digits backward

"I am going to read you a string of numbers and when I am done, you repeat them back to me backwards, in reverse order of how I read them to you. For example, if I say 7-1-9, you would say 9-1-7."

If correct, go to next string length. If incorrect, read trial 2. **One point possible for each string length.** Stop after incorrect on both trials. The digits should be read at the rate of one per second.

Months in reverse order

"Now tell me the months of the year in reverse order. Start with the last month and go backward. So you'll say December, November ... Go ahead"

1 pt. for entire sequence correct

Delayed Recall

The delayed recall should be performed after completion of the Balance and Coordination Examination.

"Do you remember that list of words I read a few times earlier? Tell me as many words from the list as you can remember in any order."

Score 1 pt. for each correct response

Balance Examination

Modified Balance Error Scoring System (BESS) testing[5]

This balance testing is based on a modified version of the Balance Error Scoring System (BESS)[5]. A stopwatch or watch with a second hand is required for this testing.

"I am now going to test your balance. Please take your shoes off, roll up your pant legs above ankle (if applicable), and remove any ankle taping (if applicable). This test will consist of three twenty second tests with different stances."

(a) Double leg stance:

"The first stance is standing with your feet together with your hands on your hips and with your eyes closed. You should try to maintain stability in that position for 20 seconds. I will be counting the number of times you move out of this position. I will start timing when you are set and have closed your eyes."

(b) Single leg stance:

"If you were to kick a ball, which foot would you use? [This will be the dominant foot] Now stand on your non-dominant foot. The dominant leg should be held in approximately 30 degrees of hip flexion and 45 degrees of knee flexion. Again, you should try to maintain stability for 20 seconds with your hands on your hips and your eyes closed. I will be counting the number of times you move out of this position. If you stumble out of this position, open your eyes and return to the start position and continue balancing. I will start timing when you are set and have closed your eyes."

(c) Tandem stance:

"Now stand heel-to-toe with your non-dominant foot in back. Your weight should be evenly distributed across both feet. Again, you should try to maintain stability for 20 seconds with your hands on your hips and your eyes closed. I will be counting the number of times you move out of this position. If you stumble out of this position, open your eyes and return to the start position and continue balancing. I will start timing when you are set and have closed your eyes."

Balance testing – types of errors

1. Hands lifted off iliac crest
2. Opening eyes
3. Step, stumble, or fall
4. Moving hip into > 30 degrees abduction
5. Lifting forefoot or heel
6. Remaining out of test position > 5 sec

Each of the 20-second trials is scored by counting the errors, or deviations from the proper stance, accumulated by the athlete. The examiner will begin counting errors only after the individual has assumed the proper start position. **The modified BESS is calculated by adding one error point for each error during the three 20-second tests. The maximum total number of errors for any single condition is 10.** If a athlete commits multiple errors simultaneously, only one error is recorded but the athlete should quickly return to the testing position, and counting should resume once subject is set. Subjects that are unable to maintain the testing procedure for a minimum of **five seconds** at the start are assigned the highest possible score, ten, for that testing condition.

OPTION: For further assessment, the same 3 stances can be performed on a surface of medium density foam (e.g., approximately 50cm×40cm×6cm).

Tandem Gait[6,7]

Participants are instructed to stand with their feet together behind a starting line (the test is best done with footwear removed). Then, they walk in a forward direction as quickly and as accurately as possible along a 38mm wide (sports tape), 3 meter line with an alternate foot heel-to-toe gait ensuring that they approximate their heel and toe on each step. Once they cross the end of the 3m line, they turn 180 degrees and return to the starting point using the same gait. A total of 4 trials are done and the best time is retained. Athletes should complete the test in 14 seconds. Athletes fail the test if they step off the line, have a separation between their heel and toe, or if they touch or grab the examiner or an object. In this case, the time is not recorded and the trial repeated, if appropriate.

Coordination Examination

Upper limb coordination

Finger-to-nose (FTN) task:

"I am going to test your coordination now. Please sit comfortably on the chair with your eyes open and your arm (either right or left) outstretched (shoulder flexed to 90 degrees and elbow and fingers extended), pointing in front of you. When I give a start signal, I would like you to perform five successive finger to nose repetitions using your index finger to touch the tip of the nose, and then return to the starting position, as quickly and as accurately as possible."

Scoring: 5 correct repetitions in < 4 seconds = 1

Note for testers: Athletes fail the test if they do not touch their nose, do not fully extend their elbow or do not perform five repetitions. **Failure should be scored as 0.**

References & Footnotes

1. This tool has been developed by a group of international experts at the 4th International Consensus meeting on Concussion in Sport held in Zurich, Switzerland in November 2012. The full details of the conference outcomes and the authors of the tool are published in The BJSM Injury Prevention and Health Protection, 2013, Volume 47, Issue 5. The outcome paper will also be simultaneously co-published in other leading biomedical journals with the copyright held by the Concussion in Sport Group, to allow unrestricted distribution, providing no alterations are made.

2. McCrory P et al., Consensus Statement on Concussion in Sport – the 3rd International Conference on Concussion in Sport held in Zurich, November 2008. British Journal of Sports Medicine 2009; 43: i76-89.

3. Maddocks, DL; Dicker, GD; Saling, MM. The assessment of orientation following concussion in athletes. Clinical Journal of Sport Medicine. 1995; 5(1): 32–3.

4. McCrea M. Standardized mental status testing of acute concussion. Clinical Journal of Sport Medicine. 2001; 11: 176–181.

5. Guskiewicz KM. Assessment of postural stability following sport-related concussion. Current Sports Medicine Reports. 2003; 2: 24–30.

6. Schneiders, A.G., Sullivan, S.J., Gray, A., Hammond-Tooke, G. & McCrory, P. Normative values for 16-37 year old subjects for three clinical measures of motor performance used in the assessment of sports concussions. Journal of Science and Medicine in Sport. 2010; 13(2): 196–201.

7. Schneiders, A.G., Sullivan, S.J., Kvarnstrom, J.K., Olsson, M., Yden, T. & Marshall, S.W. The effect of footwear and sports-surface on dynamic neurological screening in sport-related concussion. Journal of Science and Medicine in Sport. 2010; 13(4): 382–386.

Appendix I Sport Concussion Assessment Tool 3 (SCAT 3).[2]

ATHLETE INFORMATION

Any athlete suspected of having a concussion should be removed from play, and then seek medical evaluation.

Signs to watch for

Problems could arise over the first 24–48 hours. The athlete should not be left alone and must go to a hospital at once if they:

- Have a headache that gets worse
- Are very drowsy or can't be awakened
- Can't recognize people or places
- Have repeated vomiting
- Behave unusually or seem confused; are very irritable
- Have seizures (arms and legs jerk uncontrollably)
- Have weak or numb arms or legs
- Are unsteady on their feet; have slurred speech

Remember, it is better to be safe.
Consult your doctor after a suspected concussion.

Return to play

Athletes should not be returned to play the same day of injury.
When returning athletes to play, they should be **medically cleared and then follow a stepwise supervised program,** with stages of progression.

For example:

Rehabilitation stage	Functional exercise at each stage of rehabilitation	Objective of each stage
No activity	Physical and cognitive rest	Recovery
Light aerobic exercise	Walking, swimming or stationary cycling keeping intensity, 70% maximum predicted heart rate. No resistance training	Increase heart rate
Sport-specific exercise	Skating drills in ice hockey, running drills in soccer. No head impact activities	Add movement
Non-contact training drills	Progression to more complex training drills, eg passing drills in football and ice hockey. May start progressive resistance training	Exercise, coordination, and cognitive load
Full contact practice	Following medical clearance participate in normal training activities	Restore confidence and assess functional skills by coaching staff
Return to play	Normal game play	

There should be at least 24 hours (or longer) for each stage and if symptoms recur the athlete should rest until they resolve once again and then resume the program at the previous asymptomatic stage. Resistance training should only be added in the later stages.

If the athlete is symptomatic for more than 10 days, then consultation by a medical practitioner who is expert in the management of concussion, is recommended.

Medical clearance should be given before return to play.

Scoring Summary:

Test Domain	Score		
	Date:	Date:	Date:
Number of Symptoms of 22			
Symptom Severity Score of 132			
Orientation of 5			
Immediate Memory of 15			
Concentration of 5			
Delayed Recall of 5			
SAC Total			
BESS (total errors)			
Tandem Gait (seconds)			
Coordination of 1			

Notes:

CONCUSSION INJURY ADVICE

(To be given to the **person monitoring** the concussed athlete)

This patient has received an injury to the head. A careful medical examination has been carried out and no sign of any serious complications has been found. Recovery time is variable across individuals and the patient will need monitoring for a further period by a responsible adult. Your treating physician will provide guidance as to this timeframe.

If you notice any change in behaviour, vomiting, dizziness, worsening headache, double vision or excessive drowsiness, please contact your doctor or the nearest hospital emergency department immediately.

Other important points:

- Rest (physically and mentally), including training or playing sports until symptoms resolve and you are medically cleared
- No alcohol
- No prescription or non-prescription drugs without medical supervision. Specifically:
  - No sleeping tablets
  - Do not use aspirin, anti-inflammatory medication or sedating pain killers
- Do not drive until medically cleared
- Do not train or play sport until medically cleared

Clinic phone number

Patient's name

Date/time of injury

Date/time of medical review

Treatingphysician

Contact details or stamp

Appendix I Sport Concussion Assessment Tool 3 (SCAT 3).[2]

Pocket CONCUSSION RECOGNITION TOOL™

To help identify concussion in children, youth and adults

FIFA

RECOGNIZE & REMOVE

Concussion should be suspected **if one or more** of the following visible clues, signs, symptoms or errors in memory questions are present.

1. Visible clues of suspected concussion

Any one or more of the following visual clues can indicate a possible concussion:

Loss of consciousness or responsiveness
Lying motionless on ground/Slow to get up
Unsteady on feet / Balance problems or falling over/Incoordination
Grabbing/Clutching of head
Dazed, blank or vacant look
Confused/Not aware of plays or events

2. Signs and symptoms of suspected concussion

Presence of any one or more of the following signs & symptoms may suggest a concussion:

- Loss of consciousness
- Seizure or convulsion
- Balance problems
- Nausea or vomiting
- Drowsiness
- More emotional
- Irritability
- Sadness
- Fatigue or low energy
- Nervous or anxious
- "Don't feel right"
- Difficulty remembering
- Headache
- Dizziness
- Confusion
- Feeling slowed down
- "Pressure in head"
- Blurred vision
- Sensitivity to light
- Amnesia
- Feeling like "in a fog"
- Neck Pain
- Sensitivity to noise
- Difficulty concentrating

3. Memory function

Failure to answer any of these questions correctly may suggest a concussion.

"What venue are we at today?"
"Which half is it now?"
"Who scored last in this game?"
"What team did you play last week/game?"
"Did your team win the last game?"

Any athlete with a suspected concussion should be IMMEDIATELY REMOVED FROM PLAY, and should not be returned to activity until they are assessed medically. Athletes with a suspected concussion should not be left alone and should not drive a motor vehicle.

It is recommended that, in all cases of suspected concussion, the player is referred to a medical professional for diagnosis and guidance as well as return to play decisions, even if the symptoms resolve.

RED FLAGS

If ANY of the following are reported then the player should be safely and immediately removed from the field. If no qualified medical professional is available, consider transporting by ambulance for urgent medical assessment:

- Athlete complains of neck pain
- Increasing confusion or irritability
- Repeated vomiting
- Seizure or convulsion
- Weakness or tingling/burning in arms or legs
- Deteriorating conscious state
- Severe or increasing headache
- Unusual behaviour change
- Double vision

Remember:

- In all cases, the basic principles of first aid (danger, response, airway, breathing, circulation) should be followed.
- Do not attempt to move the player (other than required for airway support) unless trained to so do
- Do not remove helmet (if present) unless trained to do so.

from McCrory et. al, Consensus Statement on Concussion in Sport. Br J Sports Med 47 (5), 2013

Appendix II Pocket Concussion Recognition Tool.

Chapter 5

General Management

Jonny Gordon

5.1 Analgesia and Anesthesia

One of the most important interventions that can be made after an injury is the administration of analgesia. There are many ways in which this can be done. Having a good overall understanding of what options are available to you and **making sure you have these medications with you** is key.

5

The use of simple nonpharmacological measures such as elevation or splinting a limb injury can provide good pain relief and should not be forgotten. When preparing your kit bag, you should ideally include a selection of simple splints.

If a player presents with limb pain that is completely out of proportion to what you expect despite having received appropriate analgesia you should consider the diagnosis of either a vascular injury or possibly compartment syndrome. You should examine the player thoroughly again to ascertain whether or not either is the cause of the pain.

Similarly, someone with an increasing or disproportionate headache despite adequate analgesia should be reassessed to ensure you have not missed the diagnosis of a condition such as a subarachnoid bleed.

5.1.1 Analgesia

There is a degree of crossover between analgesia and anesthesia.

Analgesia can be defined as "loss of the sensation of pain without loss of consciousness."

Anesthesia can be defined as "loss of the sensation of pain either locally or generally with or without the loss of consciousness."

The distinction can therefore appear slightly blurred and consideration should be given to whether the condition of any player in pain will benefit from either or possibly from both treatments.

It is vital to ensure that simple measures are not overlooked. Oral administration of simple analgesics such as paracetamol is often disregarded because it is perceived to be an inferior pain killer, primarily because it is readily and cheaply available over the counter, without a prescription. However, the pain relief that can result from administering paracetamol should not be underestimated. It may need to be given in conjunction with another oral or intravenous (IV) analgesic, but even by itself it provides good pain relief and should not be overlooked (**Table 5.1**).

Analgesia can be given orally, rectally, intramuscularly (IM), or IV.

We will focus on the oral and IV routes as there is very little indication to administer analgesia by the IM route and most people with a Glasgow Coma Scale (GCS) of 15 will not tolerate medications *per rectum* (PR) when there are other options open to them.

Co-codamol 8/500 is not recommended as it provides no better analgesia than paracetamol alone but has a more significant side effect profile. (**Table 5.2**).

Nonsteroidal Anti-Inflammatory Drugs

This family of medications provides analgesic, antipyretic, and, at higher doses, anti-inflammatory properties (see, e.g., ibuprofen; **Table 5.3**).

The side-effect profile is not insignificant and a careful history should be taken to ensure there are no contraindications such as peptic ulcer disease, renal disease, or asthma. Previous sensitivity is an absolute contraindication.

Nonsteroidal Anti-inflammatory Drugs (NSAIDs) work by blocking the cyclooxygenase enzymes Cox-1 and Cox-2. These enzymes produce prostaglandins that promote pain, inflammation, and pyrexia. Cox-1 also produces prostaglandins that protect the gastric mucosa and support platelet function. When blocked, all these effects are inhibited, resulting in a decrease in inflammation, pain,

Table 5.1

Paracetamol

Use	**Mild to moderate pain**
Dose	1 g for adults or 15–20 mg/kg as a loading dose in children
Pros	Readily available and cheap; easy to administer
Cons	Significant liver and renal damage in overdose

Table 5.2

Co-codamol (30/500)

Use	**Moderate pain**
Dose	1 g for adults; not recommended in children
Pros	Very few over paracetamol alone; 30/500 (30-mg codeine phosphate and 500-mg paracetamol) will provide better analgesia than paracetamol alone
Cons	Significant side-effect profile—nausea, vomiting, dizziness constipation, and respiratory distress; possibility of dependence if overused.

Table 5.3

Ibuprofen

Use	**Mild to moderate pain**
Dose	400–600 mg up to max of 2.4 g/d (short-term use)
Pros	Comparatively safe side-effect profile; cheap and readily available
Cons	Side-effect profile increases with increasing dose as does anti-inflammatory action

and temperature. Unfortunately, they also cause an increase in gastric irritation and ulceration as well as prolonged clotting.

There is ongoing controversy about the longer-term effects that inhibiting the inflammatory process may have on the rate of healing of tissues such as muscle, ligament, and tendon. It is up to each clinician to make a personal decision based on their own experience and the available evidence, and to decide whether to prescribe these medications for athletes with acute injury.

NSAIDs can also be administered PR, IM, topically, or even IV if diluted in a significant volume of at least 500 mL for IV infusion.

The topical route is well marketed and appears to provide some analgesia although this does not appear comparable to the oral (PO) route. The side-effect profile is the same for both routes.

IM administration can be problematic and cause sterile abscesses, so it is best avoided if at all possible.

Opiates

The opiate family should be used to provide analgesia to players suffering from severe pain. The significant side-effect profile of all methods of administration of opiates should mean its use is reserved only for such patients.

Opiates can be given orally, topically, IM, or IV. In terms of management of a sporting injury, opiate administration should really be limited to the IV route, as by definition the injury will be such that control of pain is paramount and time critical. The IM route is not appropriate due to the time taken and the variability of absorption.

It is vital that a player is never left unattended once they have had an IV dose of morphine and their observations should be assessed regularly.

Respiratory and neurological depression can occur as well as hypotension and these features should be looked for and treated if they arise. More common side effects include nausea and vomiting, and an antiemetic may be required in association.

Caution should be exercised in any player with an injury requiring morphine and an associated head injury, as their conscious level may be affected and their pupils become very small (pinpoint) as a result of the drug. If administering morphine, you must have access to equipment to allow you to treat the potential complications, as well as naloxone to treat respiratory arrest.

Entonox

Nitrous oxide in a 50:50 concentration may be used to allow analgesia and sedation for procedures such as the reduction of a fracture or dislocation.

Caution should be exercised in anyone with a chest or head injury as the nitrous will preferentially diffuse into air containing spaces resulting in worsening of a pneumothorax or pneumocranium.

It is self-administered and although the player should be monitored, including their oxygen saturations, relatively few complications are encountered.

5.1.2 Anesthesia

Local anesthesia is beneficial in allowing assessment and treatment of wounds. Simple nerve blocks may also provide effective pain relief for injuries such as fractures of the femur or even of the digits. Again, having an understanding of the properties of such medications will enable you to choose the correct drug and the most appropriate method of administering it in any given situation.

Lignocaine (Lidocaine)

This is the most commonly used local anesthetic agent. It has a short time of onset and duration of action, so if used as a nerve block you may need to consider the addition of a longer-lasting agent such as bupivacaine. If large volumes are required, then the addition of adrenaline can double the quantity used.

Dose is 2 to 3 mg/kg of 1% solution. Therefore, in a 70-kg adult, the maximum dose would be about 200 mg, which equals 20 mL of 1%. The addition of adrenaline allows a maximum of 7 mg/kg to be administered. It is less painful if injected slowly and with a small caliber needle. Warming the solution also helps decrease the pain of injection. **Lignocaine does not work well when injected into or around infected wounds.**

All local anesthetics are potentially cardiotoxic and neurotoxic, and you should look out for signs of toxicity such as light-headedness, dizziness, abnormal taste, tinnitus, slurred speech, or twitching progressing to seizures. The player may not know to tell you this unless you specifically ask them.

Cardiovascular signs will vary depending on whether or not the solution has had adrenaline added. If it has, the player may develop tachycardia and hypertension. If no adrenaline is used then bradycardia with associated hypotension is more likely. Cardiovascular effects are a consequence of the anesthetic directly acting on the myocardium.

Treatment of local anesthetic toxicity is symptom dependent. Treat according to the ABCs. If the player is fitting, then use either diazepam or lorazepam to control.

Bupivacaine

This has not only a longer time of onset, but also a longer duration of action (approximately 5 hours or

so), making it good for blocks. It is more cardiotoxic than lignocaine.
The dose is the same with or without adrenaline (2 mg/kg). In a 70-kg man, administer approximately 150 mg, which is 30 mL of 0.5%.

Topical Anesthetics

These are of limited value in the pitchside setting, with the exception of amethocaine in the context of corneal abrasions. This treatment will provide almost instant pain relief, allowing assessment of the eye. It is a one-off dose as it will delay epithelial healing if used repeatedly. Effects will wear off after about 30 minutes.

5.1.3 Nerve Blocks

Femoral Nerve Block

This technique is worth noting as it will allow analgesia for anyone with a femoral fracture. It will not provide analgesia for lower-leg fractures. The block can facilitate movement of the player and application of a splint.
Dose. Dose is 10 to 15 mL of lignocaine 1% or 5 mL of lignocaine 1% + 5 mL of bupivacaine 0.5%.
Anatomy. The femoral nerve (L2–L4) is the largest branch of the lumbar plexus. It descends to the midpoint of the inguinal ligament, at which point it passes deep into the ligament and enters the femoral triangle lateral to the femoral artery, which is the most important clinical landmark. It supplies the anterior thigh muscles and the hip and knee joints, as well as providing sensation to the anteromedial thigh.
Technique. Clean the skin around the groin, then palpate the femoral artery just below the inguinal ligament. Using a green needle, inject about 1 cm **lateral** to the femoral artery pulse. Aspirate to ensure you do not enter the artery. If the player complains of paresthesia, withdraw the needle slightly and then inject. (It is important not to inject directly into the nerve.) If there is no paresthesia, then penetrate the skin to a depth of approximately 2 to 3 cm and start to inject at this point.
From this depth (1 cm lateral to the artery and 2- to 3-cm deep), inject the local anesthetic and then aim the needle slightly laterally and inject more. Ensure you continue to inject local anesthetic more superficially as you withdraw the needle.
Remember the mnemonic NAVY: from lateral to medial, Nerve, Artery, Vein, Y-fronts.

Digital Nerve Block

This is equally applicable to fingers and toes. It will provide analgesia for phalangeal fractures and dislocations and allow manipulation if necessary. It is also useful in nail and nail-bed injuries.
Dose. Dose is 1 to 2 mL of 1% lignocaine.
Anatomy. The fingers have dorsal and palmar digital nerves, while the toes have the dorsal and plantar digital nerves. The nerves can be blocked either between the metacarpals or at the proximal phalanx.
Technique. Using a 23- or 25-gauge needle, identify the bony proximal phalanx. Use a dorsal approach to inject, aiming to penetrate the skin just lateral to the bone and coming slightly medially under the bone. Aspirate to ensure no intravascular injection. Inject 0.5 to 1 mL of 1% lignocaine. Repeat on the medial side of the finger. Inject a further 0.5 mL across the dorsal aspect of the finger to ensure the dorsal nerves have been caught.

5.2 Wound Management

Wounds occur commonly in sport and their immediate management can be difficult due to the time constraints placed on the clinician to get the player back onto the field of play as soon as possible.
The initial management of all wounds should be to ensure optimum healing. This involves an adequate assessment of the depth and length of the wound, the underlying structures, and tissues affected, and the presence of debris.
Remember: If you do not look for it, you will not find it.
Good basic management involves thorough wound cleaning, usually including wound irrigation. This is far more important than the administration of antibiotics, which should rarely if ever be used as prophylaxis for infection.

5.2.1 History

How was the wound sustained? In a scalp laceration, attention should initially be paid to the cervical spine. Once the initial assessments have been made, the wound can be properly assessed.
A laceration over the knuckle with or without an underlying fracture is a common site for a fight-bite injury. It is highly prone to infection, so an honest history is vital from the player.
Tetanus status is not of great importance in the initial assessment of a player you are trying to return to the field of play but a vital medicolegal question you must document in your notes. Be aware of the immunization status of all your players.

5.2.2 Examination

- **What type of wound is it?** Most wounds will be lacerations, i.e., ragged edges caused by shearing and splitting of the tissues from blunt trauma (compare with an incised wound caused by a sharp object such as a knife). A breach of the skin overlying a fracture suggests a compound fracture.

- **What is the location of the wound?** A wound sustained over the forehead or supraorbital ridge may cause significant issues for a footballer as they are required to head the ball. An identically sized wound in the same person but over the occiput may be managed differently as it is less likely to receive further trauma during the match.
- **What are the dimensions (length and depth) of the wound?** Depth is very important as some full-thickness wounds (i.e., fully through the skin) may need to be closed in layers to ensure healing and minimize collections.
- **Are there any associated musculotendinous or neurovascular complications?**
- **Is there any foreign body contamination?** This is an exceptionally easy thing to overlook, especially in wounds that are rushed when assessed. Contaminants may come in the form of impregnated clothing such as a sock in the wound, or soil, grass, bone, or tooth.

5.2.3 Immediate Management

The best possible treatment for all but the smallest and most superficial of wounds is removal of the player from the field, ideally to an appropriately stocked treatment room. Ensure that you bring another member of staff with you if at all possible. They can then update the manager on whether you can sort the wound quickly enough to return the player or let the manager know that the player is unable to return to play.

The wound must be cleaned and explored thoroughly. The wound edges should be gently opened to allow a depth assessment to be made. This may need to be done under local anesthetic, so ensure you have documented normal sensation distal to the wound before you instil the agent.

Use saline-soaked gauze swabs to clean the wound thoroughly under direct vision. Remove and document any contaminants within the wound. A surgical scrubbing brush can be used to loosen any adherent contaminant. Irrigate the wound with sterile solution. This is the best way to ensure the wound has been properly cleaned out. A 20-mL syringe attached to a white needle can be used. After attaching the needle to the syringe, use the protective cover to gently bend the needle back and forth until it breaks at the plastic base. This will now allow a relatively high-pressure jet of sterile solution to be irrigated into the wound. In case of splashing, the operator should wear eye protection if at all possible. Refill the syringe and repeat until the wound is clean.

Bleeding points should be directly compressed for at least a minute and then reassessed. In highly vascular areas such as the scalp, lignocaine and adrenaline may be of use. If a player is bleeding from a scalp wound that cannot be controlled with the methods above, the wound can be oversewn using a large suture such as silk1–0, taking big ' bites" to pull the wound together.

Tourniquets are best avoided but can be used for a short time for the assessment of finger injuries. Cut off the small finger of a rubber glove and roll this down the finger as close to the knuckle as possible. Needle holders can then be used to clasp the rubber Rotating the needle holder will twist the rubber tighter around the finger. Use this technique for a maximum of 15 minutes before releasing and cutting the rubber away.

5.2.4 Wound Closure

Most wounds in a sporting setting are likely to be suitable for primary closure. If a wound is presented to you after more than 12 hours, do not close it; instead leave it open (after thorough cleaning) and arrange for a specialist review (no more than 48 hours later) to allow a decision on whether the wound should undergo delayed primary closure or be granulated (secondary closure). Wounds to the face and scalp may be closed up to 24 hours after they are sustained due to the excellent blood supply, but there is a significant risk of subsequent infection and wound dehiscence.

A number of options are available to close a wound (**Table 5.4**, **Table 5.5**, **Table 5.6**, **Table 5.7**). If you have not learned to suture, then do not attempt it. It is not the remit of this manual or the course to teach this skill. Instead, clean the wound, apply a dressing as best you can, and transfer the patient to the nearest emergency department.

Table 5.4

Steri-Strips	
Pros	Cheap, quick, easily to remove and reapply
Cons	Wound must be dry or the Steri-Strip will just slide off
Uses	Superficial wounds not fully through the skin
Tip	Use in conjunction with skin glue: Steri-Strips to hold wound in place and glue in between, or glue to help stick Steri-Strips onto the skin

Table 5.5

Tissue adhesive	
Pros	Cheap, quick
Cons	You only have one chance to apply, then the tissue is stuck
Uses	Superficial wounds with or without Steri-Strips
Tip	Do not use in any wound around the eye

5

Table 5.6

Sutures	
Pros	Cheap, readily available, good for closing deeper wounds
Cons	Operator dependent (more so than Steri-Strips), take longer to apply, usually needs local anesthetic, may leave poorer long-term cosmetic result compared with glue or Steri-Strips
Uses	Full-thickness wounds
Tip	Start in either the middle of the wound or at the apex

Table 5.7

Staples	
Pros	Quick, can be used without local anesthetic depending on the player
Cons	Operator dependent
Uses	Scalp wounds; do not consider in a frontal injury if returning the athlete to contact sport
Tip	Ensure you have staple remover with you in case you misplace one

Applying Vaseline, gauze swabs, and swathes of bandages to try to tamponade a wound implies that time has not been spent fully assessing the wound. It could be argued, however, that as long as there are no other clinical concerns the same wound can be formally treated at halftime or full time. While this may be appropriate if there is only a short time left to play, it is also a potentially hazardous manner to treat an individual and should not be undertaken routinely.

It could also be argued that to remove a player with a bleeding head with a view to suturing their wound and returning them to the field of play in under 5 minutes is an exceptionally tall order given that an assessment of concussion will have to be made in that time frame as well.

If the player cannot be safely returned to play within 5 minutes, they should probably not be returned at all.

5.2.5 Specific Wounds

Scalp

Scalp wounds can be closed with staples or sutures. Sutures are usually silk 1–0 to 3–0 depending on the site. Blood supply to the scalp is good, so healing time is fast, but bleeding from the wound can be a problem. The same applies to the face; however, ethilon is preferable to silk and staples are not appropriate. The higher the suture value, i.e., the thinner the material, the better the end cosmetic result.

When closing a scalp wound, attention must be paid to ensure that the galea has not been involved. The galea is a thick, tough fibrous sheet of tissue that connects the occipitofrontalis muscles. If torn or lacerated, this should be sutured to minimize the potential for infection and also to prevent cosmetic defects caused by asymmetric forehead movement as a result of disruption of the galea anchoring frontalis. This can be done by using a 3–0 suture and taking deep bites through the skin, subcutaneous tissue, and galea all in the one suture.

Hair should be cut or ointment used to pull it out of the way of the wound. It should, however, not be shaved as this increases the risk of wound infection.

Lip

Lip wounds should be assumed to be the result of the player's tooth being forced through the lip tissue from posterior to anterior. Check the teeth to ensure they are intact and that the patient has not aspirated a tooth or got one stuck in their lip.

The vermillion border must be approximated to with a gap less than 1 mm; otherwise, the resulting defect will be clearly apparent and leave an unsatisfactory cosmetic defect.

Tongue

Very rarely should this be sutured, i.e., only if there is ongoing and uncontrollable hemorrhage. If the wound is anterior, refer to a specialist for closure because of the risk of bifid tongue.

Hand

Consider a human bite in anyone with a wound over the knuckles. This will need to be explored under local anesthetic as a minimum and you should assume there is foreign body contamination (i.e., tooth) and tendinous disruption until proven after wound exploration.

Note: Assess the wound and deeper tissues with the finger in extension through to full flexion at the metacarpophalangeal joint for tendon damage.

Amoxicillin and Metronidazole should be prescribed for anyone with a human bite wound. Make a referral for assessment of hepatitis status.

Pretibial Wounds

In football, these are usually caused by an opponent's stud from their boot. The tissue in this area is usually thin and is rarely amenable to suturing. Thorough wound cleaning is absolutely vital and thereafter the best plan is usually to either close the wound with Steri-Strips or leave it to heal by secondary intention.

Infected Wounds

Infected wounds can occur despite the best surgical intervention and the highest standards of patient care. However, if you do not spend time assessing and cleaning a wound properly, it **will** become infected.

Rules of thumb:

- There is no place for routine antibiotics in the prophylactic treatment of noninfected wounds.
- You cannot spend too long cleaning or irrigating a wound.
- If you think a wound is infected, it will be. Remove sutures, Steri-Strips, or staples and accept that the wound is likely to need to heal by secondary intention. Start from scratch and thoroughly clean the wound. Unless the wound involves the face, you are likely to be surprised at how acceptable the end result actually is—however, the length of time it takes to heal can be a source of major frustration for both clinician and player.

5.2.6 Wound Dressings

The best procedure in wound treatment is to use the dressings with which you are most familiar. If you are unsure, do not guess—refer the player to hospital. Otherwise, a simple wound could be converted to a problematic wound purely because of the dressings chosen.

In simplistic terms, silicone nonadherent (silicone N/A) is one of the most useful dressing as it can be used on the vast majority of wounds, from burns through to lacerations and even infected wounds.

5.2.7 Tetanus

Most patients who have received **full vaccination** (i.e., five doses of tetanus toxoid) will be immune to tetanus.

Rules of thumb:

- If there is doubt about the player's vaccination status, refer them to hospital for tetanus toxoid with or without tetanus immunoglobulin (which will be given depending on whether the wound is tetanus prone or not).
- Also, refer the player to hospital if there is no history of tetanus immunization at all.

5.3 Kit

You must assume that the kit that you take with you will be the only kit you will be able to access. Do not assume that you will have access to other medications or kit if you are traveling away from your local venue.

There is no point taking kit that you do not feel trained or comfortable to use.

It is advisable to have a list of medications and kit and make sure that this is up to date at all times.

Think of items in terms of the following:

- Medical kit, e.g., antibiotics, inhalers (**Table 5.8**).
- Surgical kit, e.g., Steri-Strips (**Table 5.9**).
- Resuscitating kit, e.g., venflons, IM adrenaline (**Table 5.10**).

You must make sure you have access to your kit at all times. Leaving the stretcher or hard collar on the bus while the team is playing will not help your players should any of them need to be moved. The same applies to your defibrillator (**Fig. 5.1**).

In general terms, most of the kit you need should be placed at the side of the pitch and it is unlikely that you will be required to run onto the pitch with anything other than a pair of gloves and some gauze swabs. The airway and cervical spine can be controlled immediately with your hands.

Table 5.8

Medical kit	
Analgesics	Ibuprofen, Voltarol, Paracetamol Co-codamol (opiates)
Antibiotics	Penicillin, Flucloxacillin, Augmentin, Flagyl, Erythromycin
Gastrointestinal	Losec, Dioralyte, Imodium, Stemetil, Dextrose tablets
Eye	Amethocaine, Chloramphenicol, Fluorescein
Skin	Sunscreen, insect repellent, antihistamine tablets
Respiratory	Salbutamol inhaler, intramuscular adrenaline
Other	Pen torch, blood pressure cuff, stethoscope, auriscope/otoscope, sats probe, scissors

Table 5.9

Surgical kit	
Okay for hand luggage	Wound packs with plastic bowl, gauze ± plastic forceps
	Gauze swabs in sterile packs
	Sterile suture kits with forceps (toothed and nontoothed), scissors and needle holders
Must be checked (disposable suture kits are the best option when traveling, but these also must be checked)	Sharps bin
	Steri-Strips
	Sterile wound glue
	Staples
	Local anesthetic
	Wound cleaning solutions (tap water is generally fine). Volume is the key!

Note: In no way is this list intended to be exhaustive. It is suggested basic kit. The kit that you carry should only contain items with which you are fully familiar. You must also be familiar with the possible consequences of their use, both positive and negative, and be able to manage these accordingly.

Being a team doctor means that you should operate at your own level of competence. You should not attempt to do any procedure that you do not feel trained or comfortable to carry out. If you are being employed by a specific organization, ensure that both they and you are happy with the skills you can bring to the team. It may be expected that you should take a specific set of kit away with you. If you do not have the necessary skills to manage items within that kit, you must make this known rather than be criticized after the event.

Check and double-check all kit before you leave base and ensure that all drug items are within date and will stay in date for the duration of your trip. You should have a standard list of medications to take with you. Also, tailor extra medications as necessary to the individuals you travel with. If you have a duty of care to a traveling senior member of the board, then make sure you have appropriate medications to deal with any conditions they may have. Likewise, carrying drugs such as aspirin and glyceryl trinitrate (GTN) may be appropriate where the actual footballers are young, but your accompanying staff members may be older.

Keep a list of the medications you carry and the dates they expire. Keep this up to date at all times so you are aware when you need to replace them.

Controlled drugs such as morphine need to be fully accounted for and while this may be possible to do in your home country, you should always check with the rules and regulations relating to the import of this and any other medication into any country you travel to.

Table 5.10

Resuscitating kit	
Airway[a]	Nasopharyngeal airway (sizes 6 and 7) Guedel airway (sizes 3, 4, and 5) Laryngeal mask airway (sizes 4 and 5; I-gel suggested) Cervical collar (multiadjusting) Oxygen cylinder
Breathing	Bag valve mask (BVM), facemask, trauma mask Large-bore cannula, adhesive tape
Circulation	Large-bore cannula, adhesive tape such as Vecafix Blood glucose machine Automated external defibrillator (AED) Normal saline intravenous fluid and giving set

[a]Advanced airway kit is not necessary and you should only take this kit with you if you feel comfortable using it.

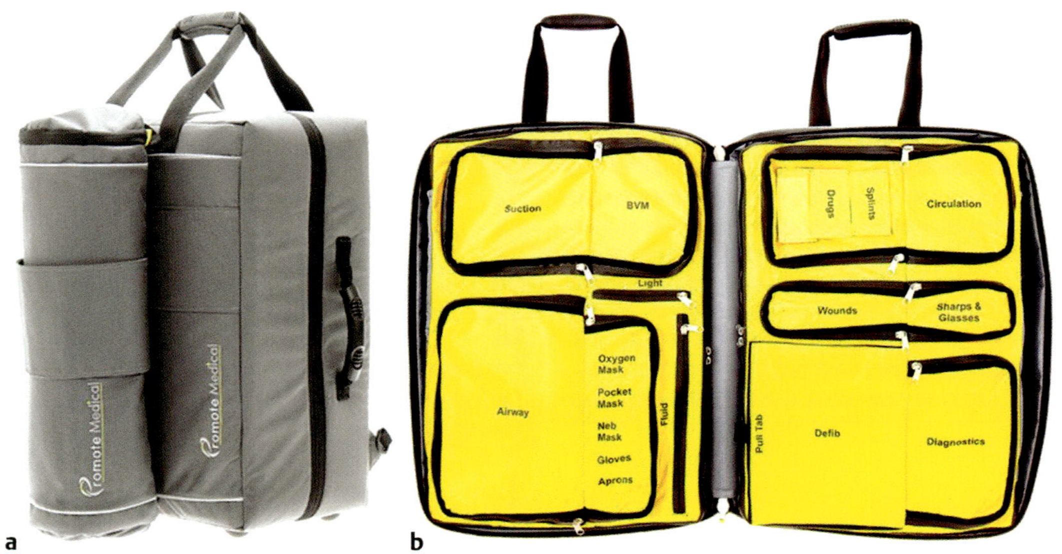

Fig. 5.1 The doctor must always carry a pitchside emergency bag with all the necessary equipment.

Chapter 6

Head Injuries

Anna Nordström

6.1 Introduction

Awareness and understanding of the consequences of head injuries and concussions has increased in football, a sport played by more than 265 million people. However, despite the best efforts of the leagues, the players, and the medical communities, incidence of head injury continues to increase. Head injuries account for 4 to 22% of all football injuries, and some studies suggest that more than half of the players in some leagues have had symptoms of concussion. The majority of concussions seem to resolve within 2 weeks of injury. However, for some players, symptoms last much longer, and returning to play with persistent symptoms increases the risk of further injury.

Concussion can be difficult to recognize and diagnose. Symptoms can be subtle, transient, and global. Often players do not report symptoms during matches or training activities. There is a common yet inaccurate perception that concussions come from head clashes and are associated with loss of consciousness. Because of this perception, many concussions remain unnoticed and unreported.

Team physicians need to be adept at evaluating, treating, and making decisions related to the short- and long-term consequences of brain trauma. Return-to-play decisions can be one of the most complex decisions and represent a dynamic evaluation of injury severity, reported symptoms, neurocognitive test results, and prior medical and concussion history.

6.2 Definitions

Concussion is a mild traumatic brain injury, frequently defined as a head injury with a temporary loss of brain function. Concussion causes a variety of physical, cognitive, and emotional symptoms, which can be subtle and difficult to recognize. The specific definition of what constitutes a concussion is still evolving. Box 6.1 shows a recently updated definition from the 4th International Conference on Concussion in Sport.

Box 6.1 Definition of Concussion from the 4th International Conference on Concussion in Sport

Concussion is a brain injury and is defined as a complex pathophysiological process affecting the brain, induced by biomechanical forces. Several common features that incorporate clinical, pathologic, and biomechanical injury constructs that may be utilized in defining the nature of a concussive head injury include the following:

- Concussion may be caused by a direct blow to either the head, face, neck, or elsewhere on the body with an "impulsive" force transmitted to the head.
- Concussion typically results in the rapid onset of short-lived impairment of neurologic function that resolves spontaneously. However, in some cases, symptoms and signs may evolve over a number of minutes to hours.
- Concussion may result in neuropathological changes, but the acute clinical symptoms largely reflect a functional disturbance rather than a structural injury and, as such, no abnormality is seen on standard structural neuroimaging studies.
- Concussion results in a graded set of clinical symptoms that may or may not involve loss of consciousness. Resolution of the clinical and cognitive symptoms typically follows a sequential course. However, it is important to note that in some cases symptoms may be prolonged.

6.3 Symptoms and Signs of Concussion

Symptoms of concussion can come and go at various times after the initial head injury and there are many additional symptoms (**Table 6.1**). Because of this, it is important to take a comprehensive approach that includes clinical examination, cognitive testing, assessment of balance and vestibular function, and symptom reports. Research shows that concussion assessments need to be repeated over time and it is best to have preseason testing for comparison with acute injuries.

Most on-field (Sport Concussion Assessment Tool 3rd Edition [SCAT3]) or follow-up concussion tools (Immediate Post-Concussion Assessment and Cognitive Testing [ImPACT], CogSport, Automated Neuropsychological Assessment Metrics [ANAM], Concussion Resolution Index [CRI], the King–Devick test) include self-reports of symptom estimation. Symptom clustering on these assessments can help provide a targeted approach to assessment,

Table 6.1

Symptoms commonly reported within 5 days of injury	
Headache	78.5%
Feeling slowed down	66.8%
Difficulty concentrating	65%
Dizziness	61.3%
Drowsiness	66.1%
Fatigue	69.2%
Visual problems	29.5%
Light sensitivity	24.3%
Memory dysfunction	55%
Balance problems	49.2%

management, and treatment. Checklists and systems usually cluster symptoms as physical, neuropsychiatric, cognitive, and sleep disturbances (**Fig. 6.1**). A player presenting with predominantly physical symptoms such as light/noise sensitivity may benefit from different treatment strategies compared to a player with mostly cognitive symptoms such as memory problems or difficulty concentrating. Careful evaluation of symptoms by category can guide the choice of management approaches, treatment plans, and rehabilitation strategies.

6.4 Causes and Mechanisms of Concussion

A concussion is caused by a direct or indirect, linear or rotational force to the head, face, or other area of the body in which the force is transmitted to the brain. The neural structures undergo a shearing strain leading to short-term neurological impairment and functional disturbances of the nervous system. In the brain, these shear forces seem to damage deep white matter tracts and microscopic injuries to the nerve axons neurons; this is also known as diffuse axonal injury. The functional disturbances, often referred to as a neurometabolic cascade, seem to cause an imbalance between energy supply and demand due to mitochondrial changes and decreased flow of blood to the brain. A corresponding increase in energy consumption occurs to reestablish homeostasis. Recovery from this imbalance requires limiting physical and cognitive activity, which may take minutes to days with subsequent symptoms lasting days to weeks.

6.5 Evaluation and Management of Concussion

Not only is it difficult to identify brain injury/concussion, but also the complex and highly individualized nature of the symptoms makes it difficult to precisely diagnose and manage. For this reason, it is important to assess individual's normal (standard) function before the injury with standardized baseline testing to use as a comparison after a potential concussion occurs (**Fig. 6.2**).

6.5.1 Baseline Testing

There are many recommendations for the use of neuropsychological assessments as part of managing concussion. Baseline testing and postconcussion testing aid the clinical decision-making process but are not the sole basis for management decisions. The ultimate return-to-play decision is a medical one in which a multidisciplinary approach should be employed.

Baseline testing is the preseason evaluation of player's cognitive function including learning, memory

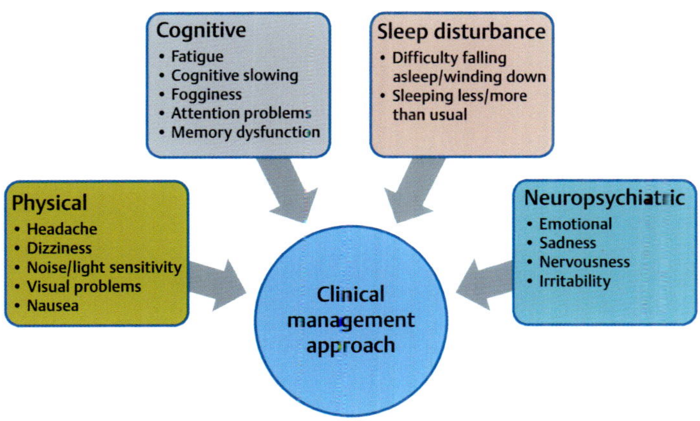

Fig. 6.1 Common symptoms associated with concussion in acute and subacute phase.

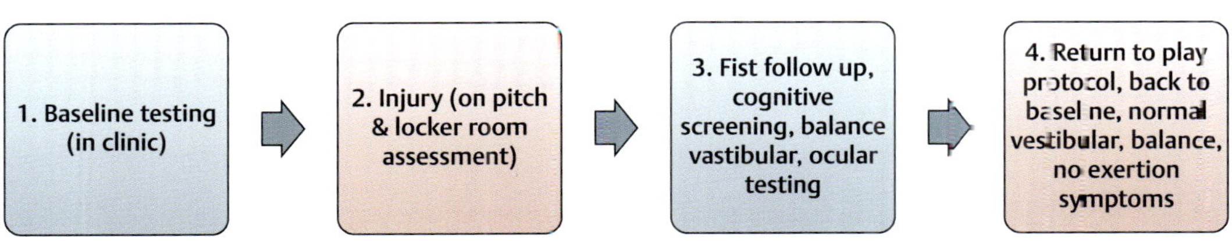

Fig. 6.2 Evaluation and management process.

skills, concentration, and problem-solving abilities. It also identifies any residual concussion symptoms from previous seasons. Baseline testing can easily be incorporated as part of the normal screening process during the preseason conditioning period. Results from baseline tests can later be compared to testing after a suspected concussion, and also to evaluate the player's recovery back to this baseline, which assists in return-to-play decisions. Comparing post-injury test scores of an individual to their own baseline test scores from before the concussion is considered best practice. Without a baseline test to use for comparison, an individual's post-injury test scores can only be compared to those of the general population.

Computerized Neuropsychological Instruments

Computerized testing of neuropsychological function decreases time spent by the clinician on preseason testing, improves test accuracy, and allows trained sports medicine clinician to interpret results without consulting a neuropsychologist. Other advantages include accessibility via internet, highly standardized test administration and scoring, the ability to compare results on multiple test forms, repeat testing, and storage of performance data for comparison purposes. The tests themselves may have higher sensitivity compared to traditional pencil-and-paper assessments.

The tests measure reaction time, memory capacity, speed of mental processing, and executive functioning. They also provide a means of assessing and storing the player's history of concussion, including number, severity, and duration of previous concussion symptoms, the age of the athlete, and any pre-existing conditions such as history of headaches, migraines, presence of attention deficit disorder (ADD/ADHD), anxiety, or any learning disabilities, including dyslexia.

There are a number of baseline tests available for sports teams to consider when implementing an overall concussion detection and management policy. To date, there is insufficient evidence to conclude that one instrument or approach is superior to another.

Immediate Post-Concussion Assessment and Cognitive Testing

ImPACT (ImPACT Applications, Inc.) is the most widely used computerized concussion evaluation system in sports today. ImPACT takes approximately 30 minutes to complete and includes a section with health history, a symptom checklist, and six neuropsychological tests, which produce four composite scores of verbal and visual memory, processing speed, and reaction time. Each composite score is compared with normative data for age and sex to provide a percentile score. The Post-Concussion Symptom Scale (PCSS), a self-reported inventory of 22 symptoms associated with concussions, is embedded into ImPACT and reported as a separate score. ImPACT test is reported to have an 82% sensitivity to detect a concussion when administered within 72 hours of trauma.

CogSport

CogSport or Axon Sports Test (CogState) is another computer-based test with good test retest reliability and a sensitive measure of cognitive recovery post-concussion. CogSport measures reaction time, accuracy to evaluate simple and complex attention, working memory, short-term memory, and ability to new learning, incidental memory, adaptive problem-solving, continuous performance, and spatial abilities. CogSport comprises a 24-item symptom checklist and 6 computerized tasks, assessing reaction time, decision-making, matching, working memory, and attention, and takes approximately 25 minutes to complete.

Automated Neuropsychological Assessment Metrics

ANAM (Vista LifeSciences) is designed to evaluate several neurocognitive domains and provide data on an individual's neurocognitive status at a point in time and changes in cognitive status over time. ANAM has been shown to be reliable and valid and measures speed and accuracy of attention, memory, and thinking abilities. ANAM includes five subset of variables such as simple reaction time, continuous performance test measuring attention and concentration, math processing measuring mental processing speed and efficiency, matching to sample measuring visual memory, and Sternberg memory measuring working memory.

Concussion Resolution Index

CRI measures reaction time and speeded decision-making. CRI has been found to be sensitive in identifying postconcussive symptoms, while remaining resistant to retest effects including changes in test performance attributed to increasing familiarity with and exposure to test. CRI consists of six subtests measuring reaction time, visual recognition, and speed of information processing.

The King–Devick Test

The King–Devick test is a fairly new promising test that has been reported to have high test–retest and inter-rater reliability, although to date, limited normative data have yet been published. The King–Devick test measures processing speed, visual tracing, and saccadic eye movements, and has been suggested to be an addition to sideline evaluation as well as baseline testing.

Paper and Pencil Test

Sport Concussion Assessment Tool 3rd Edition

A tool recommended by the latest consensus in sports concussion to aid in on-field or sideline evaluation is SCAT3, a standardized tool for evaluating athletes over the age of 13 for concussion. SCAT3 is available in an app form and also as a card to make sideline evaluation easier. SCAT3 also exists in a pediatric version (Child-SCAT3). SCAT3 can be used for baseline testing as a complement to computerized neuropsychological tests. However, to date only a few normative reference populations exists. This is however a minor detail as the players' own results, during preseason testing, should optimally be compared to the results after a sustained concussion.

SCAT3 has one observational section, one for background information, and a section of seven tests. The observational section screens for potential signs of concussion such as loss of consciousness, and amnesia. The background information section contains self-reported concussion history, risk factors for prolonged recovery, and medication history. The questions refer to known risk factors for prolonged recovery from concussion and will aid in prognosis after a sustained concussion.

The test section includes the following:

- Glasgow Coma Scale to exclude severe brain trauma.
- Maddocks five questions to test orientation and amnesia with high specificity for concussion.
- PCSS, a standardized evaluation of 22 symptoms common to concussion.
- Standardized Assessment of Concussion (SAC) to rapidly assess orientation, immediate memory, concentration, and delayed recall. *Note that the SAC cannot be substituted for comprehensive neuropsychological assessment or neurological examination beyond the field when it comes to diagnosing concussion, measuring recovery, or making return-to-play decisions.*
- Neck examination with range of motion, tenderness, and upper and lower limb sensation and strength.
- Modified balance error scoring system (BESS). double, single, and tandem leg stance, and tandem gait.
- Coordination assessment using the finger-to-nose task.

6.5.2 On-Pitch and Locker Room Acute Assessment and Management

The initial assessment is crucial for making the right call and is made when team medical personnel enter the field of play after being summoned by the referee. Fédération Internationale de Football Association (FIFA) and Union of European Football Associations (UEFA) have improved concussion management by reinforcing the team physician's role to ensure correct management of potential cases of concussions. In the event of a head injury, the referee may stop the game for 3 minutes, allowing the team physician to complete an on-field assessment. The referee may only allow the player to continue if the physician authorizes it. The following section has been divided in a short on-pitch evaluation that needs to take less than 3 minutes performed to exclude serious injuries and make a quick decision regarding risk for concussion. If a concussion is suspected, the player should be removed from the game so a more thorough assessment can be performed off-pitch.

On-Pitch Evaluation

It is difficult to rapidly assess for concussion and make a return-to-play decision in only 3 minutes. Assessment on the field can also be difficult due to the emotion and pressure around the match and because diagnostic criteria can be subtle. It is therefore advisable to use a standardized approach to clarify the acute effects of injury and establish an index of severity for increased objectivity in tracking recovery.

Exclude Acute Serious Injuries

With loss of consciousness, first evaluate **A**irway, **B**reathing and **C**irculation and perform a physical examination to rule out cervical spine or other serious injuries. Perform basic neurologic screening. If cervical spine injury is suspected or cannot be ruled out, immobilize the player's neck and transfer them to an emergency department immediately. If the player scores less than 15 on the Glasgow Coma Scale, has deteriorating mental status, or progressive worsening symptoms (for example, neurological symptoms, persistent vomiting, suspected skull fracture, or seizures), initiate urgent transportation to the nearest hospital. If none of these are present, proceed to the concussion evaluation.

Concussion Evaluation

Diagnosing concussion is straightforward if the symptoms involve loss of consciousness or if the player is obviously disoriented or anamnestic. However, in more than 90% of concussions milder deficits in cognitive function occur, making diagnosis more challenging. On approach to the player, the medical staff should observe whether there are any obvious signs of concussion, e.g., slow to get up, staggering gait, or a vacant look. A blow to the head can give a variety of symptoms that need to be checked for, including cognitive status, posture, vestibular and ocular symptoms, and abnormal behavior. If the player has had any loss of consciousness, loss of balance, motor incoordination, disorientation, confusion, amnesia, headache, or a vacant look, the player should not be allowed to return to play that day and should be referred to emergency management of hospital.

The latest consensus in sports concussion recommends using SCAT3. **Table 6.2** shows the first two tests for concussion in SCAT3. If the answer to any of these questions is yes, take the player out of play. The later sections of the SCAT3 are more suitable for off-field evaluation due to the restrictive 3-minute time frame on field.

Sideline and Locker Room Evaluation

If there is initial uncertainty over the diagnosis, before making an irreversible call for substitution or if all substitutions have been used, an expedited in-depth evaluation is possible before making the return-to-play decision. A full examination takes at least 15 minutes to perform and the recommendation is to complete the SCAT3 test in case of suspicion of concussion. If the player has any symptoms on SCAT3, the player should not be allowed to return to play.

If possible, perform concussion evaluation in the privacy of the locker room to allow for quality evaluation after the first on-pitch evaluation. If the first two sections have been used on pitch as suggested, a good strategy is to start a new SCAT3 in privacy in case there have been any deteriorations since the time of trauma. If an emergency situation has been ruled out, complete the SCAT3 evaluation starting with the seven test sections (**Table 6.2**). Complete the SCAT3 even if the call has been made to bench the player as it establishes a postinjury baseline that later can be used to track recovery and aid in evaluating if symptoms are deteriorating and a more severe injury has occurred.

A few apps are emerging as a complement to locker room screening tool with SCAT3. For example, the ImPACT system mentioned earlier also contains an app for aid in sideline evaluation measuring concentration, short-term memory, and orientation that could be useful. Another test that has developed an app for locker room screening is the previously mentioned King–Devick test evaluating visual tracking and saccadic eye movements. Neither of those app-based tests can be used for return-to-play decisions. These apps may, however, be useful in capturing important information that can assist in ongoing management and care of the suspected injury. If there is a suspicion of concussion, the player should be monitored over the next 24 hours for worsening symptoms or delayed responses. If symptoms worsen or new ones arise, the player should be referred to emergency medical care to rule out complications such as intracranial bleeding or edema. Ideally, a written notification would be given to the player with pertinent information regarding signs or symptoms that should prompt an emergency evaluation along with advice to avoid any physical or cognitive exertion that worsens or mimics signs of a concussion, including avoiding alcohol and medication such as aspirin and nonsteroidal anti-inflammatory drugs (NSAIDs) due to a theoretical risk of bleeding.

Table 6.2

On-pitch evaluation based on SCAT3 parts 1 and 2. If any of the questions have been positively answered, the player should be taken out of play

Neurological examination		
Glasgow Coma Scale less than 15	Yes	No
Deteriorating mental status	Yes	No
Potential spinal injury	Yes	No
Progressive symptoms	Yes	No
Loss of consciousness	Yes	No
Loss of memory	Yes	No
Blank or vacant look	Yes	No
Visible facial injury in combination with any of above	Yes	No
Maddocks score less than 5 points	Yes	No

6.5.3 Evaluation in Emergency Room or Doctor's Office

Despite all progress in the medical field, there is to date not a blood test, imaging, or X-ray that can detect or rule out a concussion by itself. The assessment is clinical and made by physicians trained in the identification and management of concussion. Physicians should take a careful history and assess the patient's symptoms especially whether these have improved or deteriorated since the trauma. Physical examination and additional tests, including neuroradiology, to confirm a diagnosis of concussion and exclude any structural damage to the brain should then be arranged as required.

The medical examination should include the players' medical history as well as a detailed neurological examination, including cognitive functioning, mental status, gait, and balance. Comparison can be made between the evaluation performed in the hospital setting with the initial examination made on the pitch to evaluate whether the symptoms have alleviated or worsened since the injury.

Brain Imaging

A computed tomography (CT) imaging is the recommended test for ruling out skull fracture, intracranial bleeding, or swelling of the brain within the first 48 hours of injury due to cost effectiveness and availability. CT does require exposure to radiation and cannot detect microscopic injury to the axons, which is a cause of symptoms in more severe traumatic brain injuries. Magnetic resonance imaging (MRI) is a more powerful tool for detecting microbleeds, contusions, or gliosis. While CT is the preferred test for acute trauma, it is advisable to follow it up with an MRI in a subacute phase if symptoms persist.

6.5.4 Follow-Up Evaluation and Management

Follow-up of suspected concussion should occur within 24 hours, and should include both SCAT3 and a more complete neuropsychological assessment using the tools referred to earlier in the chapter.

A player who has sustained a concussion should be instructed to rest both physically and cognitively. Cognitive rest means no reading, TV, computers, games, loud noises, or bright lights. Rest should be continued until all signs and symptoms have resolved. A gradual return-to-play protocol that will take at least 7 days to complete is the recommended management for these players (see below).

Computerized concussion screening tools may aid in discerning any lingering cognitive deficits and serial follow-up tests can be administered over days or weeks so that the medical staff can continue to track the injury. Sometimes symptoms cluster in areas such as physical, neuropsychiatric, cognitive, and sleep disturbances (see **Fig. 6.1**). Symptoms after a concussion usually linger on for 10 days, sometimes up to 3 weeks. Sometimes the symptoms persist and can develop into a postconcussion syndrome. If there is difficulty in managing symptoms or a recovery takes more than a month, refer the player to a specialized sports concussion clinic or neurology department.

Return to Play

If team medical personnel have cleared the player, a follow-up should be performed using SCAT3 and preferred cognitive tests such as ImPACT, CogSport, ANAM, CRI, or the King–Devick test. When test scores have returned to baseline and the player has been cleared, stepwise return to sport may begin.

Gradual Return-to-Play Protocol

After a player who has sustained concussion is symptom free at rest, a gradual six-step protocol as described below and shown in **Fig. 6.3** is

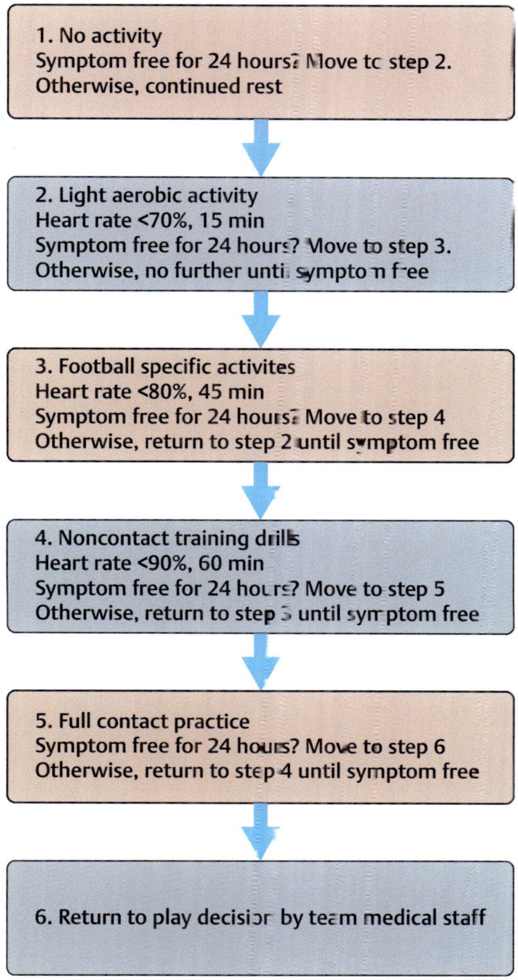

Fig. 6.3 Gradual return-to-play protocol.

recommended. This protocol includes a 24-hour gap between steps to ensure that late symptoms in response to exertion do not develop. The player can progress through each step as long as no symptoms return. If any symptoms occur, the player must return to the previous step after a minimum of a 24-hour symptom-free period and pass it without any symptoms appearing before progressing.

- *No activity.* The intention is to start a gradual return to play regardless of level or age first when the player is symptom free (without any medication) for 24 hours.
- *Light aerobic exercise.* The second step is light aerobic exercise with the purpose to increase heart rate and assess recovery. If the player experiences headache after the exercise and has a hard time to be symptom free, try to evaluate the environment in which the exertion takes place.

Management of concussions should focus on both the physical demands and the cognitive/mental exertion placed on the recovering brain. If possible, choose a location where the surrounding environment gives as little impression as possible, for example, light aerobic activity on bike in a separate room where you can control light and noise and minimize visual impressions.
- *Sport-specific exercise.* The third step is football-specific activities and more aerobic demanding activities with the purpose to add movement and assess recovery. Try to incorporate dynamic warm-ups, agility drills, and movement that challenges positional changes and the vestibular, proprioceptive, and visual systems such as burpees. Try to gradually increase the cognitive load on the player, for example, go from training in separate room to the general gym where noise, light, and movements will challenge the player. If the player manages in a quiet setting, take them outdoors. Try to integrate strength, conditioning, and balance/proprioceptive exercises.
- *Noncontact training drills.* The fourth step includes maximal exertion without contact with the purpose to add exercise and coordination together with cognitive load to assess recovery. Players can attend regular noncontact practices as a way to test them for both aerobic and cognitive exertion. Begin with reduced training volume and intensity and gradually increase load.
- *Full contact practice.* The fifth step is participation in full training including contacts and aims at restoring confidence and evaluation of functional skills by the coaching staff and allow for recovery assessment.
- The sixth step is medical clearance and return to matches.

6.6 Complications during Recovery

The following risk factors for concussion have been identified.
- A history of prior concussion.
- A greater number, severity, or duration of symptoms after a concussion.
- Low cognitive function.
- Female sex.
- Genetic predisposition.
- History of a learning disorder, ADD, migraines, or mood disorder.
- Playing certain positions.

These factors are associated with having a more protracted recovery, which may also require a more conservative management approach. If the player has symptoms after 10 days and any of the above risk factors, then refer them to a sports medicine concussion specialist, or the neurology department.

6.6.1 Symptom Management

Symptoms after a concussion usually clear during the first 10 days, although some studies suggest that 10 to 30% of individuals who sustain mild head injuries may experience symptoms and impairments for months to years. In players with prolonged recovery over a month, complete physical and cognitive rest may be unrealistic. Research suggests that active rehabilitation protocols with a subsymptom or low-level symptoms range may be a feasible way to facilitate recovery in these athletes. Thus, referring players with symptoms not resolving within 10 days to a sport concussion specialist for evaluation and active rehabilitation may be appropriate.

There is no evidence that any medication will aid recovery, although it may be considered for relief of symptoms. However, medication that could mask a deterioration in mental status within the first 24 hour should be avoided. Common symptoms to treat include headache, sleep difficulties, and depression. The team physician should go through the player's medical history to see previous and preexisting conditions and contemplate whether the symptoms could be a result of the concussion or an aggravation of a preexisting condition.

Sleep Disturbances

Sleep disturbances include difficulty falling asleep and staying asleep as well as an excessive need for sleep. Sleep disturbances can aggravate other symptoms from a concussion such as cognitive or neuropsychiatric symptoms (**Fig. 6.1**). Sleep patterns should be evaluated over time and normalized as soon as possible, striving for 9 hours a day, with no sleeping during daytime if possible. Provide normal advice regarding good sleeping hygiene. If the player has a need for daytime rest, recommend short breaks of 20 minutes and lying down to rest without sleeping to minimize impact on sleep quality during nighttime. Other recommendations include limiting TV and console/computer games.

Since players are used to high levels of physical activity during the day, inactivity in the first phase after a concussion can worsen sleep difficulties. Both pain and pain medications can also disturb sleep, as may alcohol, caffeine, or nicotine. Sleep disturbances can also mask depression or anxiety, or increase the risk of depression that is more common in individuals suffering from a concussion.

Sleep disturbances related to insomnia are usually difficult to treat with medication. Cognitive behavioral therapy for insomnia may be effective. Common pharmacological treatments are benzodiazepines in patients with underlying anxiety and nonbenzodiazepine receptor agonists such as zolpidem or eszopiclone. There is little data on treatments for excessive sleepiness. If sleep disturbances persist or are difficult to detangle from fatigue, refer the player to a concussion specialist.

Cognitive Symptoms

Fatigue can also occur and may be difficult to distinct from sleepiness. There is little data on medication for fatigue including stimulant, and players experiencing persistent fatigue should be referred to a concussion specialist or neurologist.

Neuropsychiatric Symptoms

Mood disturbances such as depression and anxiety are common symptoms after a concussion. Stress has also been linked to depressive symptoms after traumatic brain injury and may affect coping strategies and further aggravate depressive symptoms. The most commonly prescribed medication for depressive symptoms are selective serotonin reuptake inhibitors. However, there is very limited evidence of any effects of these drugs after a concussion from randomized trials. If there is a suspicion of stress or depressive symptoms, refer the player to a sports concussion specialist.

Physical Symptoms

A majority of the physical symptoms stem from the vestibular and oculomotor systems. Trauma to the brain can affect the vestibular or oculomotor systems, which affect how the brain perceives position and movement of the head; symptoms are usually described as unsteadiness, imbalance, dizziness, unsteadiness, vertigo, blurred vision, or diplopia. In this case, the brain usually relies on visual input to stabilize the head. Relying on the visual system primarily for balance often leads to fatigue, eyestrain, and tension headache.

Due to the trauma to the neck and head during the concussion, there can be a whiplash-like component resulting in cervicogenic headache. In players who have sustained concussion and have headaches, examine the cervical regions and shoulder regions, especially for players with one-sided (unilateral) headache where pain is worsened by head movements or if the player is tender to palpation in the occipital or cervical region.

Signs of autonomic dysfunction include nausea, increased heart rate, and variation in systolic blood pressure during exercise. In these cases, an exertion test with monitored heart rate and blood pressure may indicate underlying autonomic dysfunction. If there is an underlying autonomic dysregulation, active rehabilitation in the form of a subsymptom exercise protocol may be considered at a sports concussion specialist clinic.

As mentioned earlier, oculomotor or visual impairment can manifest after a concussion. A basic screening of the vestibular ocular reflex and convergence insufficiency may help in ruling out the need for specific vestibular and visual rehabilitation and can be performed by an ophthalmologist or a sports concussion specialist.

Balance symptoms are usually measured using the modified BESS in SCAT3. When balance problems are evident, the BESS containing also a foam surface could further the diagnostics.

6.6.2 Repetitive Concussions

Athletes with previous concussion are at the highest risk for new concussion especially within the first 10 days after a previous concussion; after a previous concussion, a second is three times more likely, and there may be a window of vulnerability during which a second concussion can lead to more severe traumatic brain injury or a prolonged recovery. The underlying causes for this vulnerability are unclear. If a player sustains an additional concussion within a month of a previous concussion, refer them to a sports concussion specialist as the injuries and symptoms may be more severe and can complicate recovery.

Bibliography

[1] Al-Kashmiri A, Delaney J. Head and neck injuries in football (soccer). Trauma. 2006; 8:189–195

[2] Alsalaheen BA, Mucha A, Morris LC, et al. Vestibular rehabilitation for dizziness and balance disorders after concussion. J Neurol Phys Ther. 2010; 34(2):87–93

[3] Baker JG, Freitas MS, Leddy JJ, Kozlowski KF, Willer BS. Return to full functioning after graded exercise assessment and progressive exercise treatment of postconcussion syndrome. Rehabil Res Pract. 2012; 2012:705309

[4] Barkhoudarian G, Hovda DA, Giza CC. The molecular pathophysiology of concussive brain injury. Clin Sports Med. 2011; 30(1):33–48, vii–iii

[5] Barnes BC, Cooper L, Kirkendall DT, McDermott TP, Jordan BD, Garrett WE, Jr. Concussion history in elite male and female soccer players. Am J Sports Med. 1998; 26(3):433–438

[6] Bell DR, Guskiewicz KM, Clark MA, Padua DA. Systematic review of the balance error scoring system. Sports Health. 2011; 3(3):287–295

[7] Bleiberg J, Garmoe WS, Halpern EL, Reeves DL, Nadler JD. Consistency of within-day and

across-day performance after mild brain injury. Neuropsychiatry Neuropsychol Behav Neurol. 1997; 10(4):247–253
[8] Blumbergs PC, Scott G, Manavis J, Wainwright H, Simpson DA, McLean AJ. Staining of amyloid precursor protein to study axonal damage in mild head injury. Lancet. 1994; 344 (8929):1055–1056
[9] Blumbergs PC, Scott G, Manavis J, Wainwright H, Simpson DA, McLean AJ. Topography of axonal injury as defined by amyloid precursor protein and the sector scoring method in mild and severe closed head injury. J Neurotrauma. 1995; 12(4):565–572
[10] Broglio SP, Macciocchi SN, Ferrara MS. Sensitivity of the concussion assessment battery. Neurosurgery. 2007; 60(6):1050–1057, discussion 1057–1058
[11] Brooks MA, Peterson K, Biese K, Sanfilippo J, Heiderscheit BC, Bell DR. Concussion Increases Odds of Sustaining a Lower Extremity Musculoskeletal Injury After Return to Play Among Collegiate Athletes. Am J Sports Med. 2016; 44 (3):742–747
[12] Cantu RC. Recurrent athletic head injury: risks and when to retire. Clin Sports Med. 2003; 22 (3):593–603, x
[13] Chaput G, Giguère JF, Chauny JM, Denis R, Lavigne G. Relationship among subjective sleep complaints, headaches, and mood alterations following a mild traumatic brain injury. Sleep Med. 2009; 10(7):713–716
[14] Chen JK, Johnston KM, Frey S, Petrides M, Worsley K, Ptito A. Functional abnormalities in symptomatic concussed athletes: an fMRI study. Neuroimage. 2004; 22(1):68–82
[15] Child SCAT3. Child SCAT3. Br J Sports Med. 2013; 47(5):263
[16] Collie A, Darby D, Maruff P. Computerised cognitive assessment of athletes with sports related head injury. Br J Sports Med. 2001; 35 (5):297–302
[17] Collie A, Maruff P, Makdissi M, McCrory P, McStephen M, Darby D. CogSport: reliability and correlation with conventional cognitive tests used in postconcussion medical evaluations. Clin J Sport Med. 2003; 13(1):28–32
[18] Concussion (mild traumatic brain injury) and the team physician: a consensus statement. Med Sci Sports Exerc. 2006; 38(2):395–399
[19] Covassin T, Swanik CB, Sachs ML. Epidemiological considerations of concussions among intercollegiate athletes. Appl Neuropsychol. 2003; 10(1):12–22
[20] Daniel JC, Olesniewicz MH, Reeves DL, et al. Repeated measures of cognitive processing efficiency in adolescent athletes: implications for monitoring recovery from concussion. Neuropsychiatry Neuropsychol Behav Neurol. 1999; 12(3):167–169
[21] Dashnaw ML, Petraglia AL, Bailes JE. An overview of the basic science of concussion and subconcussion: where we are and where we are going. Neurosurg Focus. 2012; 33(6) E5: E5–, 1–9
[22] Delaney JS, Lacroix VJ, Leclerc S, Johnston KM. Concussions among university football and soccer players. Clin J Sport Med. 2002; 12 (6):331–338
[23] Dziemianowicz MS, Kirschen MP, Pukenas BA, Laudano E, Balcer LJ, Galetta SL. Sports-related concussion testing. Curr Neurol Neurosci Rep. 2012; 12(5):547–559
[24] Eisenberg MA, Andrea J, Meehan W, Mannix R. Time interval between concussions and symptom duration. Pediatrics. 2013; 132(1):8–17
[25] Erlanger D, Feldman D, Kutner K, et al. Development and validation of a web-based neuropsychological test protocol for sports-related return-to-play decision-making. Arch Clin Neuropsychol. 2003; 18(3):293–316
[26] Erlanger D, Saliba E, Barth J, Almquist J, Webright W, Freeman J. Monitoring Resolution of Postconcussion Symptoms in Athletes: Preliminary Results of a Web-Based Neuropsychological Test Protocol. J Athl Train. 2001; 36 (3):280–287
[27] Fann JR, Uomoto JM, Katon WJ. Sertraline in the treatment of major depression following mild traumatic brain injury. J Neuropsychiatry Clin Neurosci. 2000; 12(2):226–232
[28] Galetta KM, Brandes LE, Maki K, et al. The King-Devick test and sports-related concussion: study of a rapid visual screening tool in a collegiate cohort. J Neurol Sci. 2011; 309 (1–2):34–39
[29] Galetta KM, Morganroth J, Moehringer N, et al. Adding Vision to Concussion Testing: A Prospective Study of Sideline Testing in Youth and Collegiate Athletes. J Neuroophthalmol. 2015; 35(3):235–241
[30] Gall B, Parkhouse W, Goodman D. Heart rate variability of recently concussed athletes at rest and exercise. Med Sci Sports Exerc. 2004; 36(8):1269–1274
[31] Goodman SR, Zimmer WE, Clark MB, Zagon IS, Barker JE, Bloom ML. Brain spectrin: of mice and men. Brain Res Bull. 1995; 36(6):593–606

[32] Greenwald BD, Kapoor N, Singh AD. Visual impairments in the first year after traumatic brain injury. Brain Inj. 2012; 26(11):1338–1359

[33] Guilleminault C, Yuen KM, Gulevich MG, Karadeniz D, Leger D, Philip P. Hypersomnia after head-neck trauma: a medicolegal dilemma. Neurology. 2000; 54(3):653–659

[34] Guskiewicz KM, Bruce SL, Cantu RC, et al. National Athletic Trainers' Association Position Statement: Management of Sport-Related Concussion. J Athl Train. 2004; 39(3):280–297

[35] Guskiewicz KM, Register-Mihalik J, McCrory P, et al. Evidence-based approach to revising the SCAT2: introducing the SCAT3. Br J Sports Med. 2013; 47(5):289–293

[36] Guskiewicz KM, Weaver NL, Padua DA, Garrett WE, Jr. Epidemiology of concussion in collegiate and high school football players. Am J Sports Med. 2000; 28(5):643–650

[37] Guskiewicz KM. Assessment of postural stability following sport-related concussion. Curr Sports Med Rep. 2003; 2(1):24–30

[38] Guskiewicz KM. Postural stability assessment following concussion: one piece of the puzzle. Clin J Sport Med. 2001; 11(3):182–189

[39] Hänninen T, Tuominen M, Parkkari J, et al. Sport concussion assessment tool - 3rd edition - normative reference values for professional ice hockey players. J Sci Med Sport. 2016; 19(8):636–641

[40] Harmon KG, Drezner JA, Gammons M, et al. American Medical Society for Sports Medicine position statement: concussion in sport. Br J Sports Med. 2013; 47(1):15–26

[41] Herring SA, Cantu RC, Guskiewicz KM, et al. American College of Sports Medicine. Concussion (mild traumatic brain injury) and the team physician: a consensus statement–2011 update. Med Sci Sports Exerc. 2011; 43(12):2412–2422

[42] Herrmann N, Rapoport MJ, Rajaram RD, et al. Factor analysis of the Rivermead Post-Concussion Symptoms Questionnaire in mild-to-moderate traumatic brain injury patients. J Neuropsychiatry Clin Neurosci. 2009; 21(2):181–188

[43] Iverson GL, Silverberg ND, Mannix R, et al. Factors Associated With Concussion-like Symptom Reporting in High School Athletes. JAMA Pediatr. 2015; 169(12):1132–1140

[44] Jeter CB, Hergenroeder GW, Hylin MJ, Redell JB, Moore AN, Dash PK. Biomarkers for the diagnosis and prognosis of mild traumatic brain injury/concussion. J Neurotrauma. 2013; 30(8):657–670

[45] Jha A, Weintraub A, Allshouse A, et al. A randomized trial of modafinil for the treatment of fatigue and excessive daytime sleepiness in individuals with chronic traumatic brain injury. J Head Trauma Rehabil. 2008; 23(1):52–63

[46] Julien JP, Mushynski WE. Neurofilaments in health and disease. Prog Nucleic Acid Res Mol Biol. 1998; 61:1–23

[47] Kontos AP, Elbin RJ, Schatz P, et al. A revised factor structure for the post-concussion symptom scale: baseline and postconcussion factors. Am J Sports Med. 2012; 40(10):2375–2384

[48] Leddy JJ, Kozlowski K, Donnelly JP, Pendergast DR, Epstein LH, Willer B. A preliminary study of subsymptom threshold exercise training for refractory post-concussion syndrome. Clin J Sport Med. 2010; 20(1):21–27

[49] Leddy JJ, Sandhu H, Sodhi V, Baker JG, Willer B. Rehabilitation of Concussion and Post-concussion Syndrome. Sports Health. 2012; 4(2):147–154

[50] Len TK, Neary JP, Asmundson GJ, Goodman DG, Bjornson B, Bhambhani YN. Cerebrovascular reactivity impairment after sport-induced concussion. Med Sci Sports Exerc. 2011; 43(12):2241–2248

[51] Ling JM, Peña A, Yeo RA, et al. Biomarkers of increased diffusion anisotropy in semi-acute mild traumatic brain injury: a longitudinal perspective. Brain. 2012; 135(Pt 4):1281–1292

[52] Lovell MR, Iverson GL, Collins MW, et al. Measurement of symptoms following sports-related concussion: reliability and normative data for the post-concussion scale. Appl Neuropsychol. 2006; 13(3):166–174

[53] Maddocks DL, Dicker GD, Saling MM. The assessment of orientation following concussion in athletes. Clin J Sport Med. 1995; 5(1):32–35

[54] Mahmood O, Rapport LJ, Hanks RA, Fichtenberg NL. Neuropsychological performance and sleep disturbance following traumatic brain injury. J Head Trauma Rehabil. 2004; 19(5):378–390

[55] Makdissi M, Davis G, Jordan B, Patricios J, Purcell L, Putukian M. Revisiting the modifiers: how should the evaluation and management of acute concussions differ in specific groups? Br J Sports Med. 2013; 47(5):314–320

[56] Maroon JC, Lovell MR, Norwig J, Podell K, Powell JW, Hartl R. Cerebral concussion in athletes: evaluation and neuropsychological testing. Neurosurgery. 2000; 47(3):659–669, discussion 669–672

6

[57] McCrea M, Guskiewicz K, Randolph C, et al. Incidence, clinical course, and predictors of prolonged recovery time following sport-related concussion in high school and college athletes. J Int Neuropsychol Soc. 2013; 19 (1):22–33

[58] McCrea M, Hammeke T, Olsen G, Leo P, Guskiewicz K. Unreported concussion in high school football players: implications for prevention. Clin J Sport Med. 2004; 14(1):13–17

[59] McCrea M. Standardized mental status assessment of sports concussion. Clin J Sport Med. 2001; 11(3):176–181

[60] McCrory P, Meeuwisse W, Johnston K, et al. Consensus Statement on Concussion in Sport: the 3rd International Conference on Concussion in Sport held in Zurich, November 2008. Br J Sports Med. 2009; 43 Suppl 1:i76–i90

[61] McCrory P, Meeuwisse WH, Aubry M, et al. Consensus statement on concussion in sport: the 4th International Conference on Concussion in Sport held in Zurich, November 2012. Br J Sports Med. 2013; 47(5):250–258

[62] Moser RS, Iverson GL, Echemendia RJ, et al. NAN Policy and Planning Committee, Donna K. Broshek, Shane S. Bush, Sandra P. Koffler, Cecil R. Reynolds, Cheryl H. Silver. Neuropsychological evaluation in the diagnosis and management of sports-related concussion. Arch Clin Neuropsychol. 2007; 22(8):909–916

[63] Nelson LD, Janecek JK, McCrea MA. Acute clinical recovery from sport-related concussion. Neuropsychol Rev. 2013; 23(4):285–299

[64] Nilsson M, Hägglund M, Ekstrand J, Waldén M. Head and neck injuries in professional soccer. Clin J Sport Med. 2013; 23(4):255–260

[65] Nordström A, Edin BB, Lindström S, Nordström P. Cognitive function and other risk factors for mild traumatic brain injury in young men: nationwide cohort study. BMJ. 2013; 346:f723

[66] Nordström A, Nordström P, Ekstrand J. Sports-related concussion increases the risk of subsequent injury by about 50% in elite male football players. Br J Sports Med. 2014; 48 (19):1447–1450

[67] Nordström A, Nordström P. Cognitive performance in late adolescence and the subsequent risk of subdural hematoma: an observational study of a prospective nationwide cohort. PLoS Med. 2011; 8(12):e1001151

[68] Nylén K, Ost M, Csajbok LZ, et al. Increased serum-GFAP in patients with severe traumatic brain injury is related to outcome. J Neurol Sci. 2006; 240(1–2):85–91

[69] Ouellet MC, Morin CM. Efficacy of cognitive-behavioral therapy for insomnia associated with traumatic brain injury: a single-case experimental design. Arch Phys Med Rehabil. 2007; 88(12):1581–1592

[70] Papa L, Edwards D, Ramia M. Exploring serum biomarkers for mild traumatic brain injury. In: Kobeissy FH, ed. Brain Neurotrauma: Molecular, Neuropsychological, and Rehabilitation Aspects. Boca Raton, FL: CRC Press; 2015:301–308

[71] Papa L, Lewis LM, Falk JL, et al. Elevated levels of serum glial fibrillary acidic protein breakdown products in mild and moderate traumatic brain injury are associated with intracranial lesions and neurosurgical intervention. Ann Emerg Med. 2012; 59(6):471–483

[72] Pelinka LE, Kroepfl A, Schmidhammer R, et al. Glial fibrillary acidic protein in serum after traumatic brain injury and multiple trauma. J Trauma. 2004; 57(5):1006–1012

[73] Piland SG, Motl RW, Ferrara MS, Peterson CL. Evidence for the Factorial and Construct Validity of a Self-Report Concussion Symptoms Scale. J Athl Train. 2003; 38(2):104–112

[74] Rahman-Filipiak AA, Woodard JL. Administration and environment considerations in computer-based sports-concussion assessment. Neuropsychol Rev. 2013; 23(4):314–334

[75] Ramont L, Thoannes H, Volondat A, Chastang F, Millet MC, Maquart FX. Effects of hemolysis and storage condition on neuron-specific enolase (NSE) in cerebrospinal fluid and serum: implications in clinical practice. Clin Chem Lab Med. 2005; 43(11):1215–1217

[76] Reddy CC, Collins M, Lovell M, Kontos AP. Efficacy of amantadine treatment on symptoms and neurocognitive performance among adolescents following sports-related concussion. J Head Trauma Rehabil. 2013; 28(4):260–265

[77] Reeves DL, Winter KP, Bleiberg J, Kane RL. ANAM genogram: historical perspectives, description, and current endeavors. Arch Clin Neuropsychol. 2007; 22 Suppl 1:S15–S37

[78] Roiger T, Weidauer L, Kern B. A longitudinal pilot study of depressive symptoms in concussed and injured/nonconcussed National Collegiate Athletic Association Division I student-athletes. J Athl Train. 2015; 50(3):256–261

[79] Scheiman M, Gallaway M, Frantz KA, et al. Nearpoint of convergence: test procedure, target selection, and normative data. Optom Vis Sci. 2003; 80(3):214–225

[80] Schreiber S, Barkai G, Gur-Hartman T, et al. Long-lasting sleep patterns of adult patients with minor traumatic brain injury (mTBI) and

non-mTBI subjects. Sleep Med. 2008; 9 (5):481–487

[81] Semple BD, Lee S, Sadjadi R, et al. Repetitive concussions in adolescent athletes - translating clinical and experimental research into perspectives on rehabilitation strategies. Front Neurol. 2015; 6:69

[82] Shan R, Szmydynger-Chodobska J, Warren OU Mohammad F, Zink BJ, Chodobski A. A New Panel of Blood Biomarkers for the Diagnosis of Mild Traumatic Brain Injury/Concussion in Adults. J Neurotrauma. 2016; 33(1):49–57

[83] Sigurdardottir S, Andelic N, Roe C, Jerstad T, Schanke AK. Post-concussion symptoms after traumatic brain injury at 3 and 12 months post-injury: a prospective study. Brain Inj. 2009; 23(6):489–497

[84] Slobounov SM, Gay M, Zhang K, et al. Alteration of brain functional network at rest and in response to YMCA physical stress test in concussed athletes: RsFMRI study. Neuroimage. 2011; 55(4):1716–1727

[85] Smits M, Houston GC, Dippel DW, et al. Microstructural brain injury in post-concussion syndrome after minor head injury. Neuroradiology. 2011; 53(8):553–563

[86] Teunissen CE, Dijkstra C, Polman C. Biological markers in CSF and blood for axonal degeneration in multiple sclerosis. Lancet Neurol. 2005; 4(1):32–41

[87] Tomberg T, Toomela A, Ennok M, Tikk A. Changes in coping strategies, social support, optimism and health-related quality of life following traumatic brain injury: a longitudinal study. Brain Inj. 2007; 21(5):479–488

[88] Vagnozzi R, Signoretti S, Cristofori L, et al. Assessment of metabolic brain damage and recovery following mild traumatic brain injury: a multicentre, proton magnetic resonance spectroscopic study in concussed patients. Brain. 2010; 133(11):3232–3242

[89] Vajtr D, Benada O, Linzer P, et al. Immunohistochemistry and serum values of S-100B, glial fibrillary acidic protein, and hyperphosphorylated neurofilaments in brain injuries. Soud Lek. 2012; 57(1):7–12

[90] Vidal PG, Goodman AM, Colin A, Leddy JJ, Grady MF. Rehabilitation strategies for prolonged recovery in pediatric and adolescent concussion. Pediatr Ann. 2012; 41(9):1–7

[91] Viola-Saltzman M, Watson NF. Traumatic brain injury and sleep disorders. Neurol Clin. 2012; 30(4):1299–1312

[92] Wilde EA, McCauley SR, Hunter JV, et al. Diffusion tensor imaging of acute mild traumatic brain injury in adolescents. Neurology. 2008; 70(12):948–955

[93] Williamson IJ, Goodman D. Converging evidence for the under-reporting of concussions in youth ice hockey. Br J Sports Med. 2006; 40 (2):128–132, discussion 128–132

[94] Xiong H, Liang WL, Wu XR. [Pathophysiological alterations in cultured astrocytes exposed to hypoxia/reoxygenation]. Sheng Li Ke Xue Jin Zhan. 2000; 31(3):217–221

[95] Yuh EL, Mukherjee P, Lingsma HF, et al. TRACK-TBI Investigators. Magnetic resonance imaging improves 3-month outcome prediction in mild traumatic brain injury. Ann Neurol. 2013; 73(2):224–235

Index

Note: Page numbers set **bold** or *italic* indicate headings or figures, respectively.